Color Atlas of Oral Diseases in Children and Adolescents

Crispian Scully

PhD, MD, MDS, FDSRCPS, FDSRCS, FFDRCSI, FRCPath
Professor of Medicine, Pathology and Microbiology
Centre for the Study of Oral Disease
University of Bristol Dental Hospital and School
Lower Maudlin Street
Bristol, UK

Richard Welbury

PhD, MBBS, FDSRCS
Regional Consultant in Paediatric Dentistry
Department of Child Dental Health
Dental Hospital and School
University of Newcastle-upon-Tyne
Framlington Place
Newcastle-upon-Tyne, UK

M WOLFE

Copyright © 1994 Mosby–Year Book Europe Limited
Published in 1994 by Wolfe Publishing, an imprint of Mosby–Year Book Europe Limited

Printed by Grafos, Arte Sobre Papel, Barcelona, Spain

ISBN 0 7234 1945 0

For full details of all Mosby–Year Book Europe Limited titles please write to Mosby–Year Book Europe Limited, Lynton House, 7–12 Tavistock Square, London WC1H 9LB, England.

A CIP catalogue record for this book is available from the British Library.

Library of Congress Cataloging-in-Publication Data has been applied for.

Contents

Preface

This book covers the presentation of the common orofacial disorders that may be seen in children and adolescents, and also includes a wide range of less common and some rare disorders. Paediatricians, General Medical Practitioners, General Dental Practitioners, Dental Specialists, Dermatologists, Oncologists, Otorhinolaryngologists and many others are called upon to diagnose and treat children with oral problems, and we hope this book will be a useful source of assistance to them.

The arrangement of such material is not without difficulties since there are inevitable overlaps. We have arranged material about the healthy mouth first and then the obviously congenital and heritable disorders. Of course, few other conditions that affect the orofacial region do not have some genetic basis. These are covered in the remainder of the atlas which outlines diseases of teeth and their sequelae; gingival and periodontal disease; mucosal disorders; salivary gland disorders; musculoskeletal disorders; and relevant other lesions. Because of the importance of child abuse, we include a separate section on physical abuse. In some areas, notably in HIV disease which can result in disease of mucosa, gingiva and salivary glands, the illustrations and text have been gathered together in the most relevant chapter. With a few exceptions we have restricted the atlas to intra-oral photographs and radiographs though, of course, the patient must always be examined and treated as a whole person. There is no especially logical classification available and therefore we have elected to arrange material alphabetically within each of these sections. The number of illustrations of any particular condition is not necessarily a reflection of the importance of the disorder. Occasional illustrations show the fingers of ungloved hands: clinicians must of course now always wear gloves during patient care.

We are grateful to our patients and to colleagues who have helped us with some material, particularly Professor Oslei Paes de Almeida (Piracicaba, Brazil), Mr Brian Avery (Middlesborough, UK), Professor Robert Berkowitz (Washington, USA), Mr N. E. Carter (Newcastle, UK), Professor A. Craft (Newcastle, UK), Dr John Eveson (Bristol, UK), Dr P. H. Gordon (Newcastle, UK), Dr Mark Griffiths (Bristol, UK), Dr John Jandinski (New Jersey, USA), Dr Jane Luker (Bristol, UK), Dr R. I. Macleod (Newcastle, UK), Professor John Murray (Newcastle, UK), Dr June Nunn (Newcastle, UK), Dr Stephen Porter (Bristol, UK), Professor Stephen Prime (Bristol, UK) and Miss C. A. Reid (Newcastle, UK). A few of the illustrations have also appeared in *A Colour Atlas of Stomatology* (C. Scully and S. Flint) and in this respect we are grateful to Martin Dunitz (London) and Dr Stephen Flint (Dublin).

We are also grateful to Mr Ni Fathers (Bristol, UK) for technical assistance, to Connie Blake (Bristol, UK) for patiently typing the manuscript, and to Dr Stephen Porter for proof-reading.

1. The Healthy Mouth

Teeth

The teeth develop from ectoderm (**1–9**). At about the sixth week of intra-uterine life the oral epithelium proliferates over the maxillary and mandibular ridge areas to form *primary epithelial bands* which project into the mesoderm, and produce a *dental lamina* in which discrete swellings appear—the *enamel organs* of developing teeth. Each enamel organ eventually produces tooth enamel, and the mesenchyme, which condenses beneath the enamel organ (actually neuroectoderm), forms a dental papilla which produces the dentine and pulp of the tooth. The enamel organ together with the dental papilla constitute the *tooth germ*, and this becomes surrounded by a mesenchymal dental follicle, from which the periodontium forms—ultimately to anchor the tooth in its bony socket.

There are 10 deciduous (primary or milk) teeth in each jaw: all are fully erupted by the age of about 3 years (**10**). The secondary or permanent teeth begin to erupt at about 6–7 years of age (**11**) and the primary teeth begin to be slowly lost by normal root resorption. However, some primary teeth may still be present at the age of 12–13 years. The full permanent dentition consists of 16 teeth in each jaw: normally, most have erupted by about 12–14 years of age but the last molars (third molars or wisdom teeth), if present, often erupt later or may impact and/or never appear in the mouth.

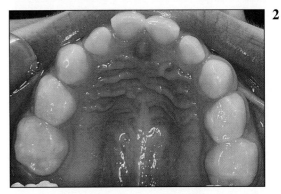

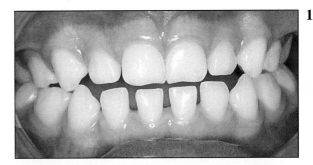

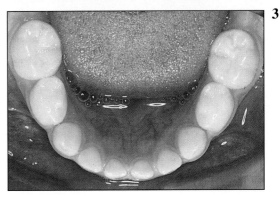

1–3 The primary dentition. Primary teeth are whiter, smaller and more bulbous than permanent teeth. Except in severely crowded mouths there is normally some spacing between primary anterior teeth.

4–6 The mixed dentition. Permanent incisors have succeeded primary incisors. The permanent molar teeth have erupted behind the primary molar teeth.

7–9 The permanent dentition. Permanent canine teeth have succeeded primary canines and permanent premolars have succeeded the primary molars.

10

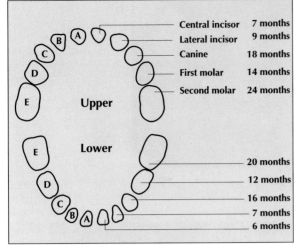

Central incisor	7 months
Lateral incisor	9 months
Canine	18 months
First molar	14 months
Second molar	24 months
	20 months
	12 months
	16 months
	7 months
	6 months

10 Eruption times: primary dentition.

11

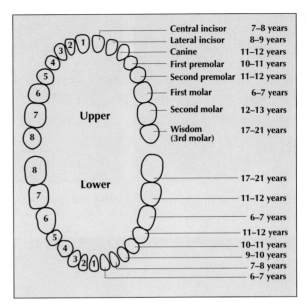

Central incisor	7–8 years
Lateral incisor	8–9 years
Canine	11–12 years
First premolar	10–11 years
Second premolar	11–12 years
First molar	6–7 years
Second molar	12–13 years
Wisdom (3rd molar)	17–21 years
	17–21 years
	11–12 years
	6–7 years
	11–12 years
	10–11 years
	9–10 years
	7–8 years
	6–7 years

11 Eruption times: permanent dentition.

Mucosa

The mucosa (**12–17**) is divided into masticatory, lining and specialised types: *masticatory mucosa* (hard palate, gingiva) is adapted to the forces of pressure and friction and keratinised with numerous tall rete ridges and connective tissue papillae and little submucosa. *Lining mucosa* (buccal, labial and alveolar mucosa, floor of mouth, ventral surface of tongue, soft palate, lips) is non-keratinised with broad rete ridges and connective tissue papillae, and abundant elastic fibres in the lamina propria.

Specialised mucosa on the dorsum of the tongue, adapted for taste and mastication, is keratinised, with numerous rete ridges and connective tissue papillae, abundant elastic and collagen fibres in the lamina propria and no submucosa. The tongue is divided by a V-shaped groove, the sulcus terminalis, into an anterior two-thirds and a posterior third. Various papillae on the dorsum include the *filiform* papillae, which cover the entire anterior surface and form an abrasive surface to control the food bolus as it is pressed against the palate, and the *fungiform* papillae. The latter are mushroom-shaped, red structures covered by non-keratinised epithelium. They are scattered between the filiform papillae and have taste buds on their surface. Adjacent and anterior to the sulcus terminalis are 8 to 12 large *circumvallate* papillae, each surrounded by a deep groove into which open the ducts of serous minor salivary glands. The lateral walls of these papillae contain taste buds.

12

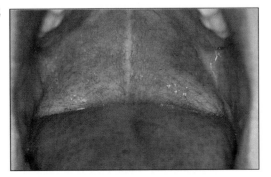

12 Normal palate (*see also* **2**, **5** and **8**).

13

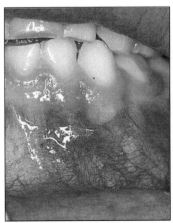

13 Normal vestibular and gingival mucosa.

14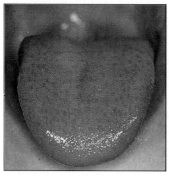

15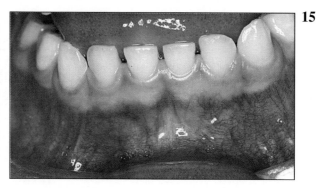

14 Normal tongue.

15 Normal mandibular labial gingivae.

16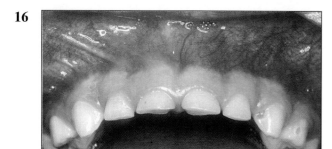
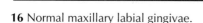

17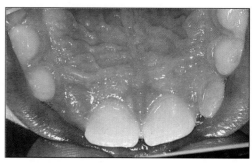

16 Normal maxillary labial gingivae.

17 Normal palatal gingivae.

The *foliate* papillae consist of 4 to 11 parallel ridges, alternating with deep grooves in the mucosa, on the lateral margins on the posterior part of the tongue. There are taste buds on their lateral walls.

The lingual tonsils are found as oval prominences with intervening lingual crypts lined by non-keratinised epithelium. They are part of *Waldeyer's oropharyngeal ring* of lymphoid tissue.

Common sensation from the mouth is conveyed by the trigeminal nerve. Taste from the anterior two-thirds of the tongue is mediated via the chorda tympani nerve and runs with the facial nerve. The glossopharyngeal nerve carries taste sensation from the posterior tongue.

Temporomandibular joints

The temporomandibular joints (TMJs) are diarthrodial joints between the condylar fossae in the temporal bones, and the mandibular condyles. Masticatory movements are controlled by the medial and lateral pterygoid muscles; the masseters; the temporalis muscles; and the mylohyoid and digastric muscles.

Salivary glands

The major salivary glands are the parotid, submandibular and sublingual glands, but minor glands are scattered throughout the oral cavity, particularly in the lower lip and palate. The secretions from the different glands differ from each other—for example, the submandibular saliva has far more mucus than does the parotid. Secretion is controlled via the glossopharyngeal (parotid) or chorda tympani (submandibular/sublingual) nerves. Normally, clear saliva can be expressed from the major ducts, or stimulated with citric acid and, at rest, there is a pool of clear saliva in the floor of the mouth. A 'dental' mirror slides easily over the oral mucosa.

2. Congenital and Heritable Disorders

Amelogenesis imperfecta

Amelogenesis imperfecta is the term applied to a number of rare genetically determined disorders of enamel formation. Multiple inheritance patterns are recognised and the incidence is of the order of 1 in 14,000. Both primary and permanent dentitions are affected. Three major categories exist:

Hypoplastic type—thin enamel of normal calcification (**18**). This includes a spectrum of disorders that may range from a localised pitting defect in enamel to a general diminution of enamel formation. In the generalised form the teeth are smaller with lack of interproximal contacts.

Hypocalcified type—enamel of normal thickness but of low radiodensity and low mineral content (**19**). This shows a great variability and the enamel of the cervical portion of the teeth is often more highly mineralised. The affected enamel is soft and is quickly lost, exposing the dentine.

Hypomaturation type—the radiodensity of enamel approaches that of dentine and easily chips away from dentine (**20, 21**). The enamel has a characteristic mottled brown–yellow–white appearance. One fairly common sub-type is known as 'snow-capped teeth', in which varying proportions of enamel in the incisal or occlusal aspects of the crowns have an opaque white appearance.

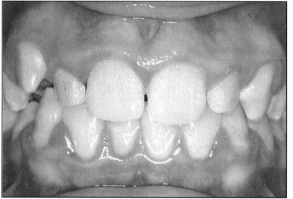

18 Random pitted autosomal dominant type of amelogenesis imperfecta.

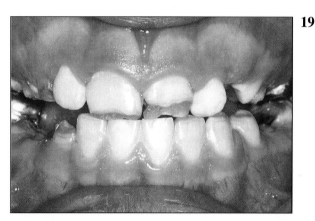

19 Hypocalcified autosomal dominant type of amelogenesis imperfecta.

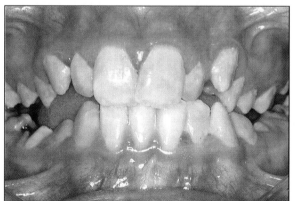

20 Pigmented hypomaturation autosomal recessive type of amelogenesis imperfecta.

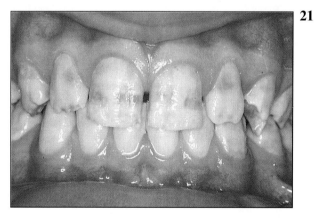

21 Hypomaturation autosomal recessive type of amelogenesis imperfecta.

Abnormal labial fraenum

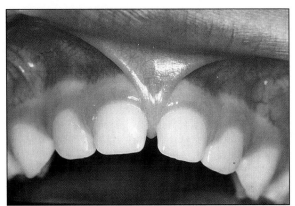

A labial maxillary fraenum (**22**) may occasionally be associated with spacing between the central incisors—a maxillary median diastema. The fraenum may need to be removed in the permanent dentition before the diastema can be closed by orthodontic means.

22 Fleshy labial frenum with a broad attachment extending to the gingival margin.

Ankyloglossia (tongue tie)

Ankyloglossia (tongue tie) affects up to 1.7% of children (**23**). It is usually a congenital anomaly of little consequence, and does not interfere with speech. A recent report shows an increased incidence in the babies of cocaine-addicted mothers. The main consequence of ankyloglossia is difficulty in using the tongue to cleanse food away from the teeth and vestibules (**24**).

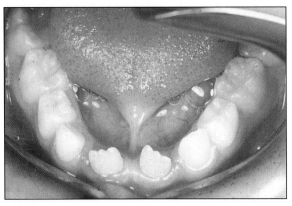

23 Tongue tie showing the lingual frenal attachment extending to the tip of the tongue preventing significant tongue protrusion.

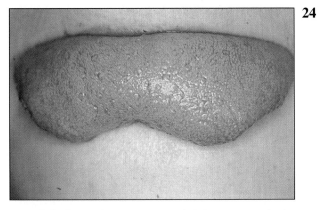

24 Ankyloglossia showing impaired ability to protrude the tongue.

Apert's syndrome (acrocephalosyndactyly)

Craniosynostosis (a high steep forehead), ocular hypertelorism and an antimongoloid slope to the eyes are characteristics of both Apert's and Crouzon's syndromes (**25**). Apert's syndrome also involves progressive synostosis of bones in the hands, feet and vertebrae as well as ankylosis of joints (**26**). Palatal anomalies are common in Apert's syndrome, and one-third of patients have cleft palate. Maxillary hypoplasia is seen.

Crouzon's syndrome is discussed on p. 18.

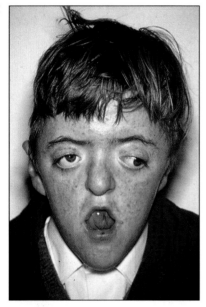

25 Apert's syndrome demonstrating the characteristic facial features.

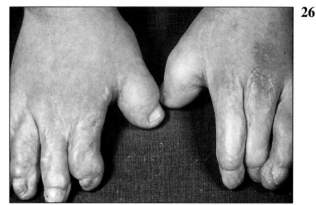

26 Digital anomalies in Apert's syndrome.

Cerebral palsy

There are no oral changes specific to cerebral palsy but there may be bruxism, malocclusion, and oral disease as a consequence of plaque accumulation (inflammatory periodontal disease), high sugar intake (caries), or medication (e.g. phenytoin-induced gingival hyperplasia if there is epilepsy) (**27**).

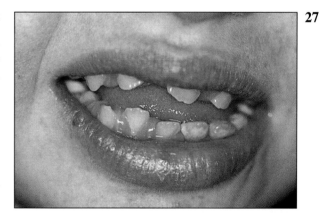

27 Cerebral palsy, showing calculus on left mandibular teeth, and phenytoin-induced gingival hyperplasia.

Cherubism (familial fibrous dysplasia)

Cherubism is the term given to a familial type of fibrous dysplasia which typically affects the angles of the mandible to produce a cherubic appearance (**28**).

Cherubism is an autosomal dominant trait, and presents particularly in males, usually after the age of 4–5 years.

Plain radiographs show multilocular radiolucencies and expansion of the mandible (**29**). The swellings increase in size and then usually regress, at least partially, at puberty. Occasionally the maxillae are involved. Submandibular lymph node enlargement can occasionally occur.

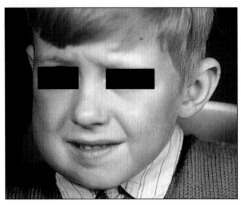

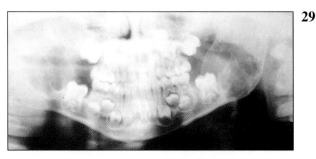

29 Pan–oral view demonstrating multilocular radiolucencies in the angles and ascending rami of the mandible of a patient with cherubism.

28 Cherubism, showing mandibular swellings especially prominent on the right.

Chondroectodermal dysplasia (Ellis–van Creveld syndrome)

Dwarfism (**30**), polydactyly, ectodermal dysplasia affecting nails and teeth (**31**), multiple fraenae and hypoplastic teeth characterise this syndrome (**32**).

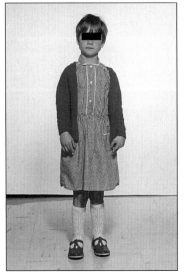

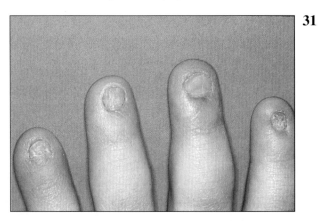

30 Chondroectodermal dysplasia: affected children are of small stature and often there is a marked genu valgum deformity.

31 Dysplastic nails in chondroectodermal dysplasia.

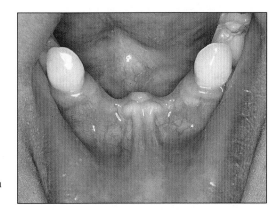

32 The lower jaw in chondroectodermal dysplasia demonstrating hypodontia and high fraenal attachments.

Clefting disorders

Bifid or cleft uvula (**33**) is a fairly common minor manifestation of cleft palate but of little consequence, though an associated submucous cleft may cause speech impairment.

Cleft lip and palate (**34–36**) are more common together than is cleft lip alone. The cleft is on the left in over 60% of patients. There is familial tendency when one parent is affected and the risk to a child is about 10%. Cleft lip and palate are, in about 20% of cases, associated with anomalies of head and neck, extremities, genitalia or heart and some cases are associated with various syndromes.

Isolated cleft palate is especially associated with Down's syndrome, Pierre Robin syndrome, Treacher Collins syndrome and Klippel–Feil syndrome.

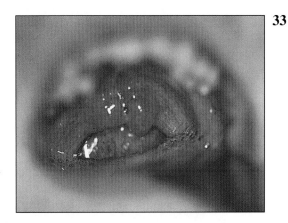

33 Bifid uvula—which may be associated with a submucous cleft.

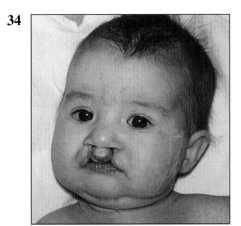

34 Bilateral cleft lip.

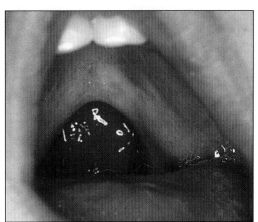

35 Isolated cleft of the posterior palate.

36

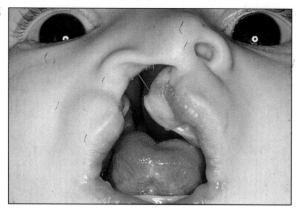

36 Cleft lip and palate.

Cleidocranial dysplasia (cleidocranial dysostosis)

Cleidocranial dysplasia is an inherited defect of membrane bones, often an autosomal dominant trait. Defects involve mainly the skull and clavicles. Persistence of the metopic suture gives rise to a vertical midline furrow in the forehead with frontal bossing (**37**). The sutures are also still open and multiple wormian bones evident in the occipito-parietal region.

The clavicles are hypoplastic or aplastic and when the patient attempts to bring the shoulders forward and together, can almost approximate them (**38**). Pelvic anomalies may be seen and kyphoscoliosis is common. The midface is hypoplastic. The dentition may be disrupted because of multiple supernumerary teeth and impactions. Radiography shows multiple unerupted and impacted teeth (**39, 40**). Dentigerous cysts commonly form.

37

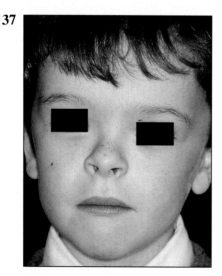

37 Hypertelorism in cleidocranial dysplasia.

38

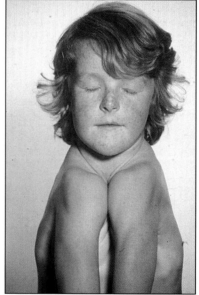

38 Absence of clavicular development allows the shoulders to be approximated in cleidocranial dysplasia.

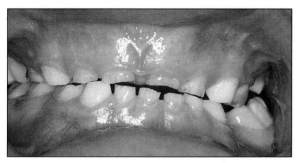

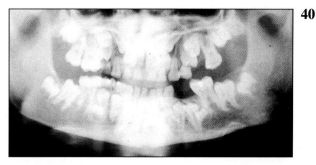

39 A 14-year-old patient with cleidocranial dysplasia, showing retention of the primary dentition.

40 The pan-oral view of the patient in **39** showing the presence of unerupted supernumerary and normal permanent teeth.

Congenital immunodeficiencies

Chronic oral candidosis, which may present as thrush and/or angular stomatitis, is an early and prominent feature in cell-mediated (T-cell) immune defects, and there is a predisposition to recurrent lesions of herpes simplex and varicella-zoster virus (**41, 42**).

Chronic mucocutaneous candidosis (CMC) is a heterogeneous group of syndromes characterised by cutaneous, oral and other mucosal candidosis, usually from early life. One variant, candidosis-endocrinopathy syndrome (Well's type 3 CMC), also includes hypoparathyroidism (with dental defects) and often hypoadrenocorticism (**43–46**), hypothyroidism and diabetes mellitus. *Candida albicans* is the usual cause of candidosis, but *C. tropicalis, C. parapsilosis, C. guilliermondii* and *C. krusei* may also be implicated. The white plaques eventually become widespread, thick and adherent, and the tongue fissured.

In CMC, candidosis involves both skin and nails in varying severity (**44**).

Granulomas may be seen in one variant of CMC (diffuse type 2). These patients also have chronic oral candidosis (**45**), and candidosis may affect the larynx and eyes.

Type 1 CMC has a familial pattern, an early onset and may have associated iron-deficiency anaemia and post-cricoid webs.

There are many other primary immune defects known. Some are barely compatible with life. Di George syndrome has additional profound defects such as cardiovascular defects: others have profound immunodeficiencies.

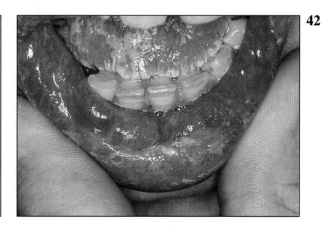

41 Severe herpes labialis in a child with a congenital T-lymphocyte defect.

42 Oral candidosis (thrush) in a congenital T-cell immune defect.

43

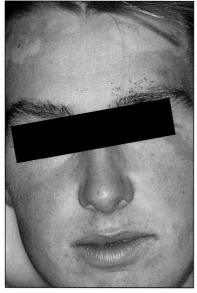

44

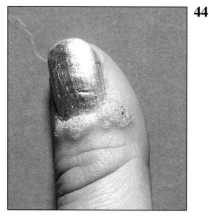

44 Nail involvement is common in chronic mucocutaneous candidosis.

43 Hyperpigmentation due to Addison's hypoadrenocorticism, and vitiligo, in a boy with candidosis-endocrinopathy syndrome.

45

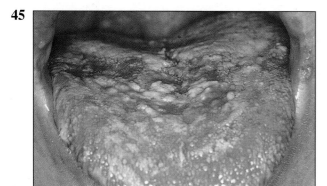
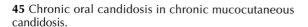

46

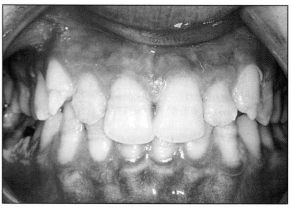

45 Chronic oral candidosis in chronic mucocutaneous candidosis.

46 Chronological hypoplasia of the anterior teeth in chronic mucocutaneous candidosis.

Wiskott–Aldrich syndrome is a rare immune deficiency syndrome with thrombocytopenia and eczema. It may be associated with oral petechiae, oral ulceration (**47**), premature tooth loss and/or large pulp chambers.

Chronic granulomatous disease (CGD) is predominantly a sex-linked leukocyte defect in which neutrophils and monocytes are defective at killing catalase-positive micro-organisms and presents typically with cervical lymph-node enlargement and suppuration. Recurrent infections in early childhood may result in enamel hypoplasia, and there is also a predisposition to oral ulceration and periodontal destruction (**48**). Other types of neutrophil defect also predispose to mouth ulcers and accelerated periodontitis (*see* p. 76). Severe infections in the neonate can disturb odontogenesis, causing enamel hypoplasia. In the past, tetracycline treatment caused tooth discolouration.

Sex-linked panhypoimmunoglobulinaemia (Bruton's syndrome) affects males almost exclusively, presents mainly with recurrent pyogenic respiratory infections, and may predispose to mouth ulcers.

Selective IgA deficiency is the most common immunoglobulin deficiency, and the main primary (genetically determined) immune defect. Some patients are healthy but others, particularly those who also lack IgG$_2$, suffer recurrent respiratory infection, autoimmune disorders and atopy. Many have mouth ulcers, and there *may* be a reduced protection against dental caries.

47

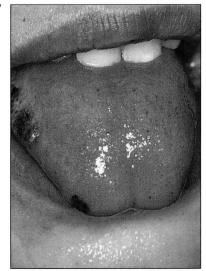

48

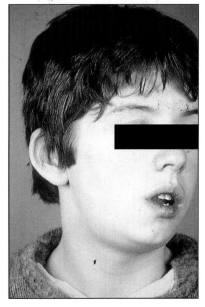

47 Oral purpura in the Wiskott–Aldrich syndrome.

48 Submandibular lymphadenitis in chronic granulomatous disease.

Congenital epulis (granular cell myoblastoma)

Congenital epulis is a rare benign swelling on the alveolus in an infant (**49**). There is a female predominance. It is probably a reactive mesenchymal lesion, usually presenting as a pedunculated firm pink swelling.

Congenital epulis is a benign tumour whose natural history may be of spontaneous regression. If there are feeding or breathing difficulties it can be excised.

49

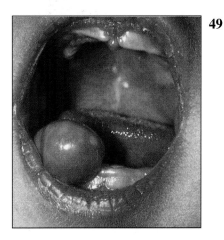

49 Congenital epulis arising from the mandibular ridge in a 7-day-old child.

Cowden's syndrome (multiple hamartoma and neoplasia syndrome)

This is an autosomal dominant condition of multiple hamartomas, with a predisposition to tumours in adult life, particularly carcinomas of breast, thyroid and colon. Papular oral lesions are common (**50**). Other oral lesions may include fissured tongue, hypoplasia of the uvula, and maxillary and mandibular hypoplasia.

Large numbers of papillomatous lesions are seen on the skin, especially over the neck, nose and ear (**51**). Mucocutaneous lesions often precede the appearance of malignant disease elsewhere.

Other manifestations of Cowden's syndrome may include small keratoses on the palms and soles, mental handicap and motor incoordination.

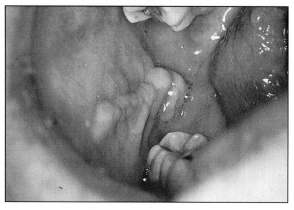

50 Oral papular lesions in Cowden's syndrome.

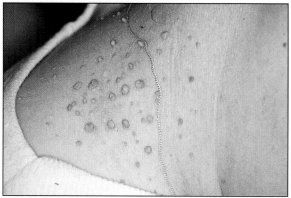

51 Papillomatous skin lesions in Cowden's syndrome.

Crouzon's syndrome (craniofacial dysostosis)

Craniosynostosis, ocular hypertelorism (**52**) and proptosis are characteristics of Crouzon's syndrome. Plain radiography shows craniosynostosis, abnormal skull morphology and pronounced digital impressions ('copper-beaten skull'). Teeth may be missing, peg-shaped or enlarged.

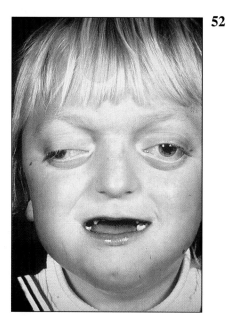

52 Crouzon's syndrome showing pronounced hypertelorism.

Cystic fibrosis

This is the commonest cause of chronic suppurative lung disease of children in the UK. It is an autosomal recessive condition with a frequency of 1 in 2,000 births. It affects many exocrine and mucus secreting glands, the primary abnormality involving defective cell membrane transport. Sweat glands, salivary glands and pancreas produce abnormal secretions resulting in duct obstruction. Salivary glands may swell. A defect in ciliary action leads to recurrent chest infections, chronic productive cough, halitosis, chest deformity, finger clubbing (**53**) and poor growth. Central cyanosis is often present .

Due to the recurrent chest infections requiring many courses of antibiotics and the development of antibiotic resistance, the use of tetracyclines may be unavoidable. The teeth may then be affected by tetracycline staining (**54**).

 53

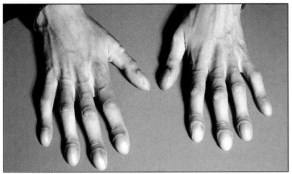

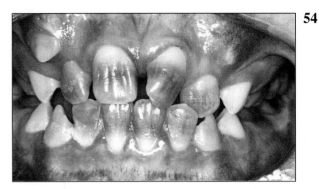 **54**

53 The hands of a patient with cystic fibrosis, demonstrating cyanosis and finger clubbing.

54 The teeth of the patient with cystic fibrosis, demonstrating tetracycline staining.

Dentinogenesis imperfecta

Dentinogenesis imperfecta (**55–60**) is an autosomal dominant condition (incidence 1:8000) in which the dentine is abnormal in structure and hence translucent.

Three types exist: type I (associated with osteogenesis imperfecta); type II (hereditary opalescent dentine); and type III (brandywine type).

55
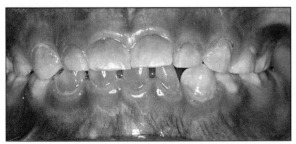

56
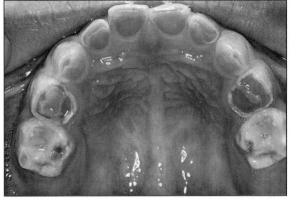

55, 56 Dentinogenesis imperfecta at age 4 years. There has been loss of enamel from the primary incisors, canines and first molars. There is early loss of enamel on the second primary molars.

The dental findings in types I and II are similar: primary teeth are more severely affected than permanent. In the permanent dentition, the teeth that develop first are generally more severely affected than those which develop later. The teeth are translucent and may vary in colour from grey to blue or brown. The enamel is poorly adherent to the abnormal underlying dentine and easily chips and wears. The crowns of the teeth are bulbous with pronounced cervical constriction, and the roots are short and fracture easily. There is progressive obliteration of pulp chambers and root canals with secondary dentine. Periapical radiolucencies are not uncommon.

Type III is an extreme variation, recognised in the primary dentition where the teeth have a 'shell-tooth' appearance, and multiple pulpal exposures are common.

57
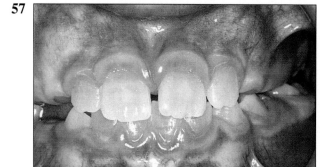

58
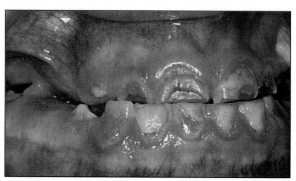

58 With unprotected posterior occlusion there is rapid loss of face height and attrition of permanent incisors.

57 Dentinogenesis imperfecta: when the permanent incisors erupt they are of normal length and contour.

59
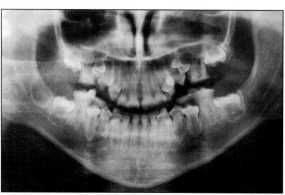

60
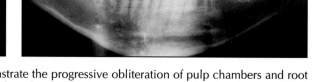

59, 60 These pan-oral views taken 3 years apart demonstrate the progressive obliteration of pulp chambers and root canals characteristic of dentinogenesis imperfecta. Onlays have been placed on the premolars and molars to prevent loss of tooth substance.

Down's syndrome

Down's syndrome (**61–63**) is a trisomic chromosome anomaly usually involving chromosome 21, in most instances affecting children of elderly mothers. There is a typical mongoloid appearance. Brachycephaly and short stature are prominent features, there are anomalies of many organs, and virtually all patients are mentally handicapped. A fairly characteristic, though not pathognomonic, feature is the presence of white spots (Brushfield spots) around the iris. Other characteristic features are a single palmar crease (simian crease) and clinodactyly of the fifth finger.

Patients with Down's syndrome have multiple immune defects and are predisposed to acute leukaemia.

Blepharitis, keratitis, upper respiratory and other infections are common.

Cheilitis and cracking of the lips may be seen, possibly because of mouth-breathing. Macroglossia and fissured tongue are also common and the midface is often hypoplastic with palatal anomalies.

Cleft lip and palate are more prevalent in Down's syndrome than in the general population.

Early loss of teeth is a feature, not only because of poor oral hygiene in many patients, but also because the teeth have short roots and there may be rapidly destructive periodontal disease.

61

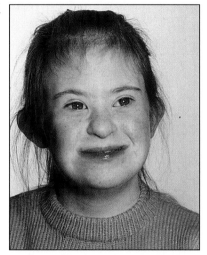

61 The characteristic facies of Down's syndrome.

62

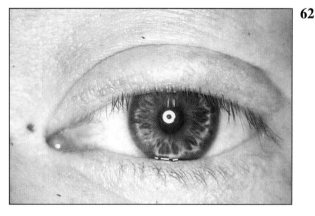

62 Brushfield spots in the iris are fairly characteristic of Down's syndrome.

63

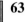

63 Hypoplasia of teeth, and periodontitis, are often associated with Down's syndrome.

Ectodermal dysplasia

Hypohidrotic ectodermal dysplasia, the most common variant, is usually a sex-linked disorder, characterised by sparse hair (hypotrichosis), absent sweat glands (hypohidrosis) and consequent fever. There may be respiratory infections, absent teeth (hypodontia) and sometimes frontal bossing (**64–69**). Patients are otherwise well and mentally normal.

There is usually hypodontia rather than anodontia, and the few teeth that are present are often of simple conical shape and erupt late. The lower third face height may therefore be reduced. Dry mouth predisposes to caries.

Rare varieties include an autosomal dominant variety (the 'tooth and nail' type), characterised by hypodontia and hypoplastic nails, and a sub-type in which teeth are normal (hypohidrotic ectodermal dysplasia with hypothyroidism).

64

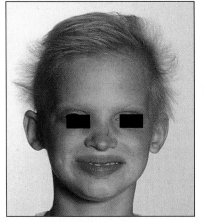

64 Characteristic facial appearance of sex-linked hypohidrotic ectodermal dysplasia (HED).

65

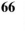

65 Xeroderma in hypohidrotic ectodermal dysplasia.

66

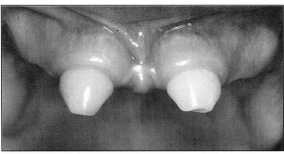

66 Severe hypodontia in sex-linked HED. The primary canines are retained but there is absence of all the permanent teeth.

67

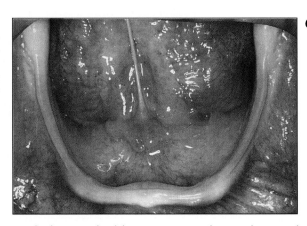

67 The lower arch of the patient in **66**: there is absence of all permanent teeth.

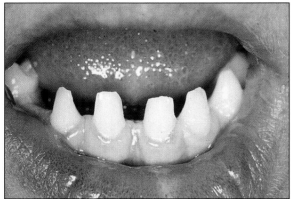

68 Hypodontia and conical teeth in HED.

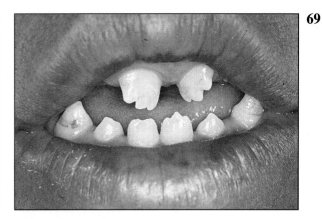

69 Dental anomalies in HED.

Ehlers–Danlos syndrome

Ehlers–Danlos syndrome is a group of inherited disorders of collagen, usually inherited as autosomal dominant traits (**70–73**). Hypermobility of joints is common (*see* p. 118), the skin is soft, extensible and fragile, purpura is common in some types and there may be other defects, such as mitral valve prolapse.

The teeth may be small with abnormally shaped roots and multiple pulp stones, and type VIII Ehlers–Danlos syndrome is associated with early onset periodontal disease.

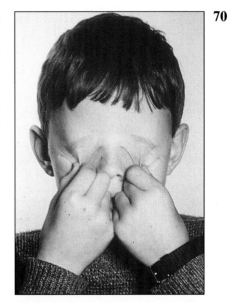

70 Hyperelasticity of the skin in Ehlers–Danlos syndrome.

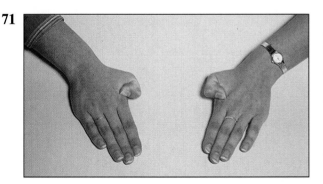

71 Hypermobility of the joints in Ehlers–Danlos syndrome.

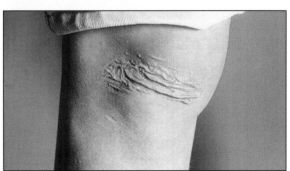

72 Due to the hyperelasticity of the skin, healing of skin lacerations over joints in Ehlers–Danlos syndrome can result in a very fine papyraceous scarring as shown here. This easily breaks down, and these lesions are best treated by a period of joint immobilisation.

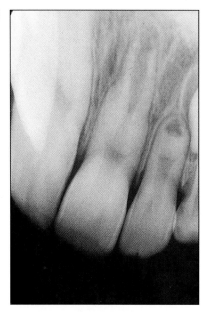

73 Premature apical closure, cessation of root growth and intrapulpal calcification in Ehlers–Danlos syndrome.

Epidermolysis bullosa

Epidermolysis bullosa is a group of rare inherited disorders of skin and mucosa, mostly characterised by vesiculation at the epithelial basement membrane zone in response to minor trauma, and consequent scarring (**74–76**). In most forms, bullae may be seen in the mouth. Bullae appear early in life, often precipitated by suckling, and break down to persistent ulcers that eventually heal with scarring. The tongue becomes depapillated and scarred. Oral lesions are seen rarely in the non-scarring simplex type of epidermolysis bullosa, in which the vesiculation is intra-epithelial.

Enamel hypoplasia may be seen, and, in view of the fragility of mucosa, oral hygiene tends to be neglected with subsequent caries and periodontal disease. Squamous cell carcinoma is a rare complication.

Scarring with the dystrophic form affects the extremities, including the nails.

An acquired form of epidermolysis bullosa (epidermolysis bullosa acquisita) is a chronic blistering disease of skin and mucosae, with autoantibodies to type VII procollagen of epithelial basement membranes.

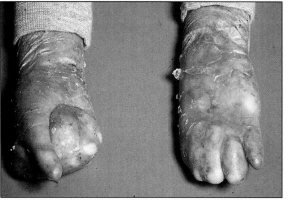

74 The hands in epidermolysis bullosa—the result of repeated epidermal breakdown and scarring.

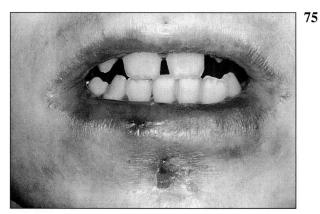

75 Scarring of the lower lip as a result of repeated bullae formation in epidermolysis bullosa.

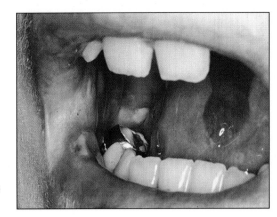

76 Intraoral bullae demonstrating the extremely fragile mucosa in epidermolysis bullosa.

Epiloia (tuberous sclerosis, Bourneville–Pringle disease)

Tuberous sclerosis is an autosomal dominant condition of mental handicap, epilepsy, and skin lesions, possibly related to a defect on chromosome 9. Most patients are both mentally handicapped and prone to seizures. Cerebral calcifications are seen on radiography (**77**).

Angiofibromas, typically seen in the nasolabial fold, are pathognomonic, can be severely disfiguring and may involve other sites, such as the chin (adenoma sebaceum) (**78**). Fibrous plaques on the forehead, 'shagreen patches' elsewhere, and hypopigmented 'ash leaf' patches seen on the trunk (**79**) are other cutaneous features. Subungual fibromas are another pathognomonic feature (**80**) and may be seen with longitudinal ridging of the nails.

Patients may also have cardiac rhabdomyomas or renal harmartomas (cysts or angiomyolipomas).

Papilliferous oral mucosa lesions may be seen and pit-shaped enamel defects are a feature (**81**). Occasional patients may have phenytoin-associated gingival enlargement.

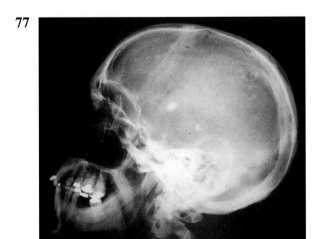

77 Cerebral calcifications in epiloia (tuberous sclerosis).

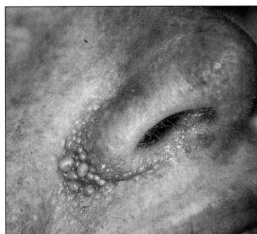

78 Adenoma sebaceum in epiloia.

79

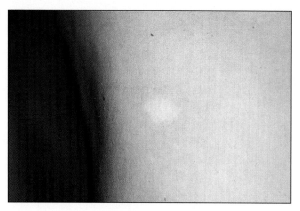

80

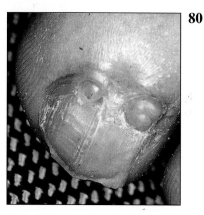

79 'Ash leaf' depigmentation in epiloia.

80 Subungual fibromas in epiloia.

81

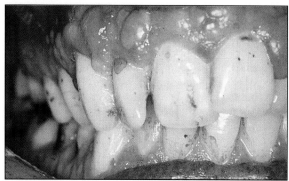

81 Gingival fibrous plaques and pitting hypoplasia of the tooth enamel in an adolescent with epiloia.

Erythema migrans (geographic tongue, benign migratory glossitis)

Erythema migrans (**82**) is a common benign condition (affecting up to 1.5%) of unknown aetiology, in which the filiform papillae desquamate in irregular demarcated areas. Patients with a fissured (scrotal) tongue often have erythema migrans. Occasionally, similar lesions may appear elsewhere on the oral mucosa, and *rarely* there is an association with pustular psoriasis.

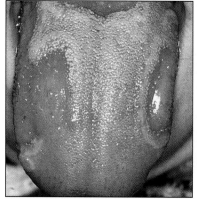

82

82 Erythema migrans (geographic tongue, benign migratory stomatitis).

Fallot's tetralogy

About 10 % of all congenital heart defects and 66 % of all cyanotic congenital heart defects are due to Fallot's tetralogy. The condition involves ventricular septal defect, pulmonary stenosis, right ventricular hypertrophy and dextroposition of the aorta. There is significant right-to-left shunting of blood, resulting in central cyanosis (**83**).

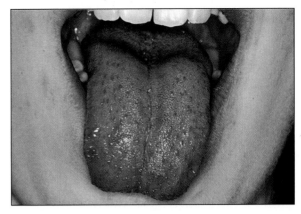

83

83 Central cyanosis of the lips and tongue in Fallot's tetralogy.

Fissured tongue (scrotal or plicated tongue)

Fissured tongue is a common developmental anomaly, affecting about 1% of children, that may appear after puberty. It is of little significance, though often associated with erythema migrans (**84**).

Fissured tongue is, however, one feature of Melkersson–Rosenthal syndrome (*see* p. 35) and is found more frequently than normal in Down's syndrome (*see* p. 21) and psoriasis.

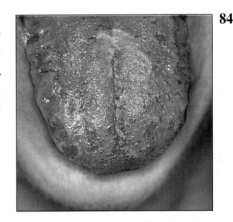

84

84 Fissured tongue, also showing erythema migrans.

Gingival cysts in neonates

Small white nodules are extremely common on the alveolar ridge and midline palate of the newborn. Sometimes termed Epstein's pearls or Bohn's nodules (**85**), they usually disappear spontaneously by rupturing or by involution within a month or so. There may be an association of gingival cysts with milia (superficial epidermal inclusion cysts).

Oral cysts are otherwise rare in neonates, although cysts may present at the base of the tongue where they can cause airway obstruction.

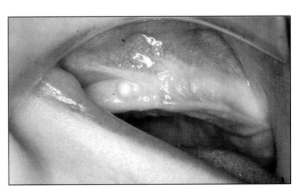

85

85 Epstein's pearls (gingival cysts) in a young infant.

Gingival fibromatoses

86

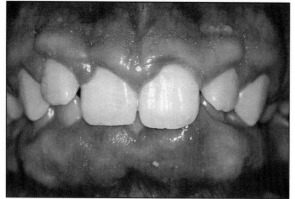

86 A mild form of hereditary gingival fibromatosis.

Hereditary gingival fibromatosis is a familial condition, in which generalised gingival fibromatosis often associated with hirsutism usually becomes most apparent at the time teeth are erupting (**86**). There are occasional associations with epilepsy, sensorineural deafness and some rare syndromes such as Laband syndrome (**87, 88**), in which there are skeletal anomalies.

87

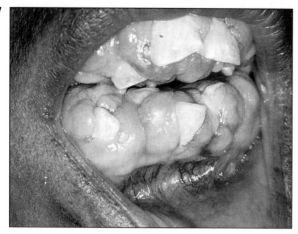

87 Pronounced gingival fibrous hyperplasia in Laband syndrome.

88

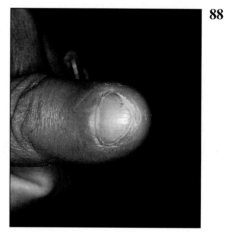

88 Digital anomalies in Laband syndrome.

Goldenhar's syndrome (oculo-auriculo-vertebral dysplasia)

In Goldenhar's syndrome, defects of the eye, ears and vertebrae are associated with orofacial, cardiac, respiratory, renal, gastrointestinal and nervous system abnormalities (**89, 90**).

Orofacial manifestations include unilateral facial hypoplasia, zygomatic, temporal, and maxillary hypoplasia, aplasia or hypoplasia of mandibular ramus and/or condyles with absence of the glenoid fossae, and flattening of the gonial angles. Macrostomia, high palate, cleft lip and palate, palate and tongue muscle hypoplasia and/or paralysis, bifid tongue, bifid uvula, double lingual fraenum, enlarged philtrum, and hypodontia may also be seen. There may also be agenesis of the ipsilateral parotid salivary gland and aberrant salivary gland tissue.

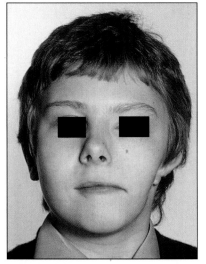

89

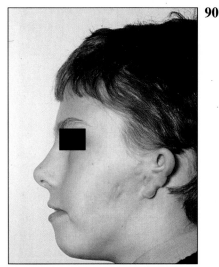

90

89 Goldenhar's syndrome demonstrating unilateral facial hypoplasia with failure of development of the external auditory meatus, canal and pinna of the ear. Accessory auricular appendages have been surgically removed.

90 Goldenhar's syndrome.

Gorlin's syndrome (Gorlin–Goltz syndrome, multiple basal cell naevi syndrome)

Gorlin's syndrome is an autosomal dominant condition of multiple basal cell naevi (**91, 92**) with odontogenic keratocysts and other features. Frontal and parietal bossing and a broad nasal root give the typical facial appearance.

Multiple basal cell naevi, often with milia, appear in childhood or adolescence (**91**), mainly over the nose, eyelids and cheeks. Only about 50% of patients have significant numbers of naevoid basal cell carcinomas and only rarely are the lesions aggressive. Pits may be seen in the soles or palms. Occasionally, basal cell carcinomas arise in these pits.

Keratocysts develop mainly in the mandible and during the first 30 years of life. Cleft lip and/or palate are seen in about 5%.

Calcification of the falx cerebri is a common feature, occurring in over 80% of patients. There are many skeletal anomalies, but bifid ribs, kyphoscoliosis and other vertebral defects are common.

Medulloblastomas and other brain tumours have been reported in several patients, as have a range of neoplasms of other tissues, especially cardiac fibromas.

Other occasional associations include pseudo-hypoparathyroidism and diabetes mellitus.

91

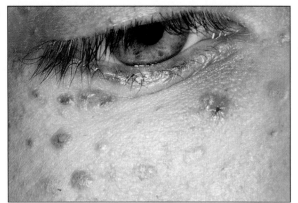

92

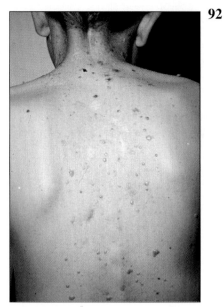

91 Basal cell naevi in Gorlin's syndrome.

92 Multiple basal cell naevi on the back of a boy with Gorlin's syndrome.

Haemangioma

Haemangiomas (**93–97**) are fairly common hamartomas in the mouth, especially on the lip and, less commonly, the tongue.

93

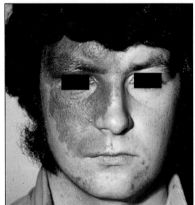

94

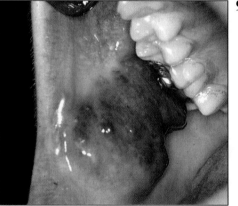

95

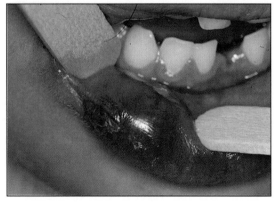

93 Haemangiomas affecting the skin may also affect the intraoral tissues and the alveolar bone. Dental instrumentation and tooth extraction can cause significant haemorrhage.

94 Haemangioma of the buccal mucosa and cheek in the patient in **93**.

95 Haemangioma in the lower lip.

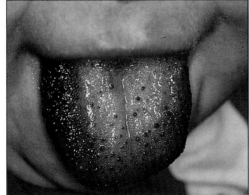

96 Haemangioma infiltrating the whole tongue.

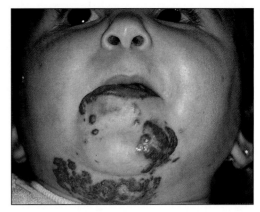

97 Haemangioma involving lip and skin.

Haemophilias

The haemophilias do not predispose to spontaneous gingival haemorrhage, oral petechiae or ecchymoses but any breach of the mucosa, especially tooth extraction, can lead to persistent bleeding that is occasionally fatal (**98**). One danger is that haemorrhage into the fascial spaces, particularly from surgery in the lower molar region, can track into the neck and constrict the airway. Haemorrhage after extraction can be controlled with clotting factor replacement, use of antifibrinolytics such as tranexamic acid, and desmopressin.

Tooth eruption and exfoliation of primary teeth are usually uneventful but, occasionally, there can be a small bleed into the follicle.

HIV infection may manifest orally in patients given infected blood transfusions or blood products before suitable screening and heat-treatment became available.

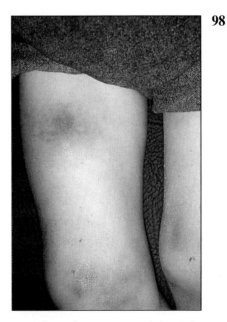

98 A large haematoma of the right thigh as a result of persistent bleeding into the muscle in haemophilia A.

Hypoparathyroidism

In congenital hypoparathyroidism, there may be pronounced hypoplasia of the teeth, shortened roots and retarded eruption (**99**).

Rare patients with candidosis-endocrinopathy syndrome and with Di George syndrome also have chronic mucocutaneous candidosis as well as hypoparathyroidism.

Acquired hypoparathyroidism produces facial tetany (Chvostek's sign) but no oral manifestations.

In pseudohypoparathyroidism (**100–104**) there are elfin facies, short stature, short metatarsals and metacarpals, calcified basal ganglia and enamel hypoplasia. Parathyroid hormone is secreted, but the end organs are unresponsive and there is also an association with other endocrine disorders, particularly hypothyroidism.

99

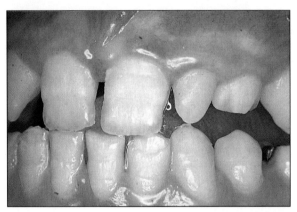

99 Enamel hypoplasia in congenital hypoparathyroidism.

100

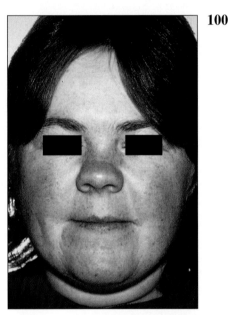

100 The characteristic somatic features of round 'elfin facies' and short stocky neck in pseudohypoparathyroidism.

101

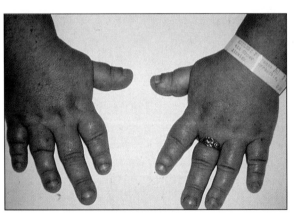

101 The small dumpy hands of the patient in **100**.

102

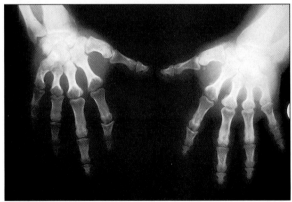

102 The radiographs reveal shortening of all metacarpals and distal phalanges in pseudohypoparathyroidism.

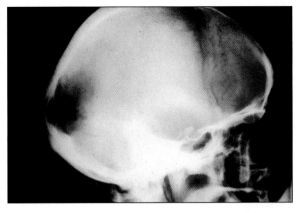

103 The lateral skull of the same patient (**100**) showing calcification within the basal ganglia.

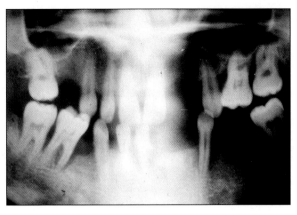

104 A pan-oral view of the same patient (**100**) showing a decimated teenage dentition with pulp stones in the upper left and lower right first permanent molars.

Incontinentia pigmenti (Bloch–Sulzberger disease)

Incontinentia pigmenti is a type of ectodermal dysplasia. It is a rare dominant disorder seen virtually only in females. Pigmented, vesicular or verrucous skin lesions are seen, often with mental handicap and visual defects.

Most patients have dental anomalies and both dentitions may exhibit anomalies. Hypodontia (**105**), conical teeth and delayed eruption (**106**) are the usual oral features.

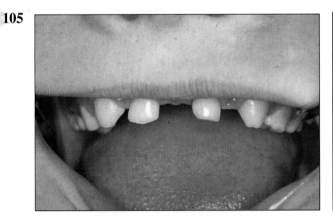

105 Incontinentia pigmenti showing hypodontia.

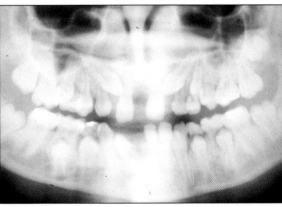

106 Incontinentia pigmenti showing missing lateral incisors.

Lip pit

Commissural lip pits (**107**) are uncommon blind epithelial-lined developmental anomalies inherited as an autosomal dominant trait. Usually of no consequence, they may be associated with pre-auricular pits. Pits may also be paramedian on the vermilion, may exude mucus, and are most often associated with cleft lip or palate.

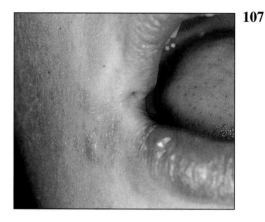

107

107 Congenital lip pit.

Lymphangioma

Lymphangioma (**108–110**) is an hamartoma of lymphoid tissue, most common in the anterior tongue or lip, typically with a 'frogspawn' appearance.

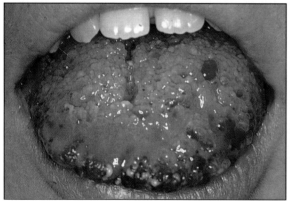

108

108 Lymphangioma involving the tongue.

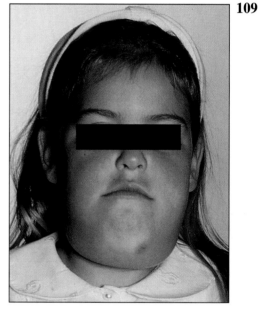

109

109 Large submental lymphangioma.

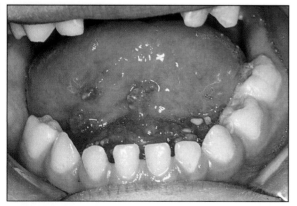

110

110 Same patient as in **109** showing lymphangioma under the tongue.

Melkersson–Rosenthal syndrome

Melkersson–Rosenthal consists of facial paralysis, facial swelling (**111**), fissured tongue and plicated mucosal swelling (**112**). Not all patients have every component of the syndrome, which is closely related to orofacial granulomatosis and oral Crohn's disease (*see* p. 89).

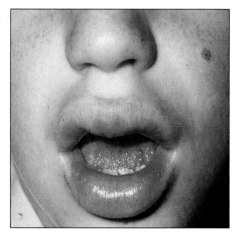

111

111 Facial oedema, involving the lips especially, in Melkersson–Rosenthal syndrome.

112

112 Plication and swelling of the midline palatal mucosa in Melkersson–Rosenthal syndrome.

Mucopolysaccharidosis (Hurler's syndrome or gargoylism)

Deficiency of mucopolysaccharidases leads to the accumulation of mucopolysaccharides (glycosaminoglycans) and one of a number of syndromes characterised by dwarfism, hirsutism, coarse features (**113**), and macroglossia, often with mental handicap, deafness, cardiac failure and corneal clouding. Hurler's syndrome is the most common of these disorders. It manifests in early childhood with deteriorating mental and physical development.

The head is large with premature closure of sagittal and metopic sutures. The pituitary fossa is boot- or slipper-shaped.

Hepatosplenomegaly causes abdominal swelling, and umbilical hernia is common.

Characteristic 'claw hand' occurs because the joints cannot be fully extended. There are also flexion contractures in many other joints.

There are frequent upper respiratory infections, cardiomegaly and murmurs. Delayed or incomplete eruption of teeth and radiolucent lesions around the crowns of the lower second molars may occur as well as temporomandibular joint anomalies (**114**).

113

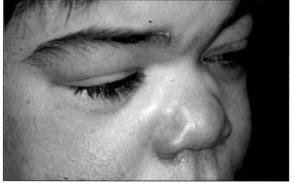

113 Coarse facial features and saddle nose in Hurler's syndrome.

114

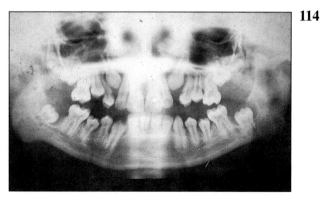

114 Radiolucencies around the second molar crowns, and temporomandibular joint anomalies, in Hurler's syndrome.

Mucosal neuromas

Neuromas in lips and tongue (**115**) may be part of a Multiple Endocrine Adenomatosis (Type IIB) syndrome which may include medullary thyroid carcinoma, phaeochromocytoma and parathyroid hyperplasia.

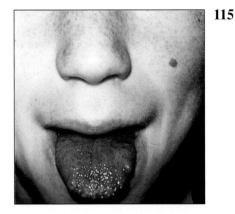

115

115 Multiple neuromas on the tongue in a patient with multiple endocrine adenomatosis syndrome (MEA type IIB).

Natal and neonatal teeth

Rarely, teeth are present at (natal), or soon after (neonatal), birth (**116, 117**), and have been described even at 26 weeks' gestation. The incidence is from 1 in 700 to 1 in 6, 000 births. They may cause no problems but can ulcerate the tongue (Riga–Fede disease) (**117**), or the mother's breast if the infant is suckling. Usually the teeth involved are lower incisors of the normal primary dentition; in less than 10% they are supernumeraries. Rarely, there are associations with Ellis–van Creveld syndrome; pachyonychia congenita; Hallermann–Streiff syndrome, or steatocystoma multiplex.

If there are problems from natal teeth, radiographs should be taken. Extractions are best restricted to those teeth that are supernumeraries or are very loose and in danger of being inhaled.

116

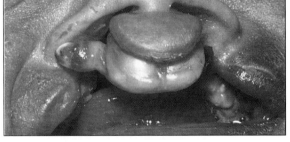

116 Two natal teeth, one on each side of the premaxilla, in a newborn baby with bilateral cleft lip and palate.

117

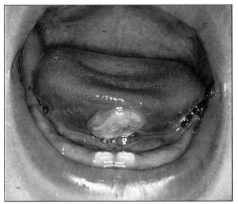

117 Ulceration of tongue caused by neonatal teeth.

Odontodysplasia

This condition is a true odontodysgenesis imperfecta, affecting all histologic elements of the dental organ but usually involving only adjacent teeth in one segment of a dental arch (**118, 119**).

Both primary and secondary teeth can be affected. Affected teeth have been termed 'ghost teeth' because of their lack of density and faded character in standard radiographs.

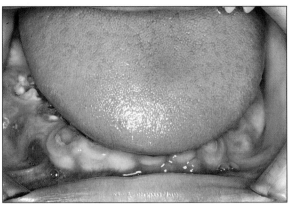

118 Odontodysplasia affecting the mandible. There are retained primary tooth remnants and buccal abscesses.

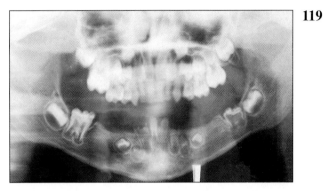

119 A pan-oral view of the same patient as in **118** taken 3 years later. The lower second permanent molars appear to be developing relatively normally.

Oral-facial-digital syndrome

Multiple fibrous bands may be associated with cleft or lobulated tongue in oral-facial-digital syndrome (OFD). In OFD type I, which is seen only in girls, there is also clinodactyly, cleft palate and sometimes renal defects. OFD type II (**120**) is less severe but there is often also conductive deafness.

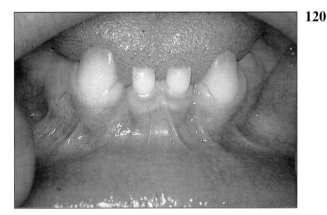

120 Hypodontia and multiple fibrous bands in oral-facial-digital syndrome type II (Mohr's syndrome). The primary incisors are retained.

Osteogenesis imperfecta (fragilitas ossium)

Osteogenesis imperfecta is a group of rare disorders in which a defect in type 1 collagen leads to fragile bones that fracture with minimal trauma (**121**). There are several sub-types varying in severity: features may include otosclerosis, blue sclerae, hypermobile joints, cardiac valve defects (mitral valve prolapse or aortic incompetence), vertebral collapse and subsequent pareses, and dentinogenesis imperfecta.

The primary dentition may be affected by dentinogenesis imperfecta in some types of osteogenesis imperfecta (**122**), but the permanent dentition is often unaffected.

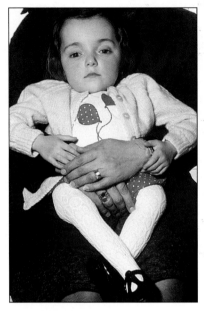

121 Osteogenesis imperfecta.

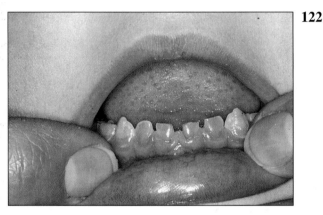

122 Teeth of patient in **121** showing dentinogenesis imperfecta.

Papillon–Lefévre syndrome

Papillon–Lefévre syndrome is a rare, genetically-linked disorder manifesting with pre-pubertal periodontitis (**123**) in association with palmar-plantar hyperkeratosis (**124**). Virtually all primary teeth are involved and most are lost by the age of 4 years. The permanent teeth are often lost by the age of 16 years.

Hyperkeratosis usually affects the soles more severely than the palms. The dura mater may be calcified, particularly the tentorium. The choroid can also be calcified.

A rare variant of the Papillon–Lefévre syndrome includes arachnodactyly and tapered phalanges as well as the above features.

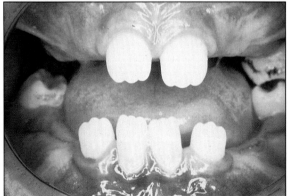

123 Periodontitis in Papillon–Lefévre syndrome.

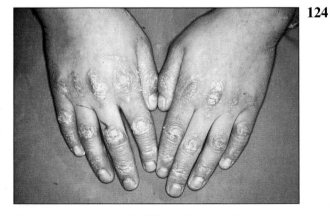

124 Hyperkeratosis in Papillon–Lefévre syndrome.

Patau's syndrome

Cleft lip (often bilateral) and cleft palate with micrognathia are orofacial features of trisomy 13 (**125**).

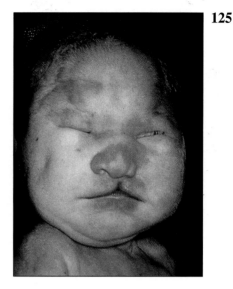

125

125 Patau syndrome showing cleft lip.

Pierre Robin syndrome

The Robin syndrome (or sequence) is severe congenital micrognathia with cleft palate (**126**). The Robin sequence may be seen in Stickler syndrome (a disorder of type II collagen) and in foetal alcohol, methadone or foetal hydantoin syndromes. There may be glossoptosis and respiratory embarrassment. Episodic dyspnoea is often evident from birth. There may also be congenital cardiac anomalies and mental handicap.

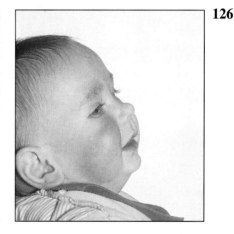

126

126 Robin sequence.

Racial pigmentation

There is no direct correlation between skin colour and gingival pigmentation (**127**) which may be seen in coloured races and others, such as those of southern European descent.

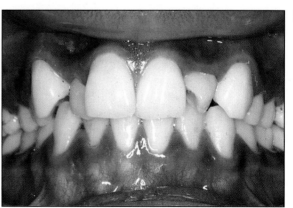

127

127 Racial pigmentation.

Rett's syndrome

Rett's syndrome (**128, 129**) is a recently recognised disorder seen only in females and characterised by progressive neurological disorder, loss of purposeful hand use, and acquired microcephaly. Constant bruxism is a conspicuous feature.

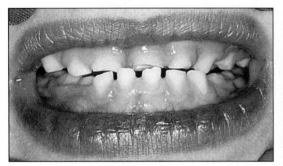

128

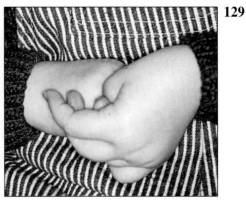

129

128 Pronounced attrition due to bruxism in Rett's syndrome.

129 Wringing of hands in Rett's syndrome.

Soto's syndrome

Soto's syndrome consists of advanced height and bone maturation dating from infancy, mental deficiency and unusual craniofacial appearance (**130**). The facies is characterised by macrocrania with dolichocephaly and ocular hypertelorism with antimongoloid obliquity of palpebral fissures (**131**). The frontal hairline is often receded.

High arched palate, precocious dental eruption and mandibular prognathism are the oral manifestations (**132**).

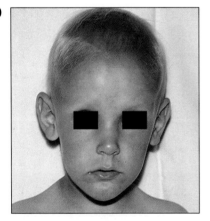

130

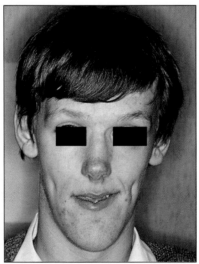

131

130 An infant aged 4 years with Soto's syndrome.

131 The same patient as in **130** at age 17 years. There is pronounced macrocrania and dolichocephaly with mandibular prognathism.

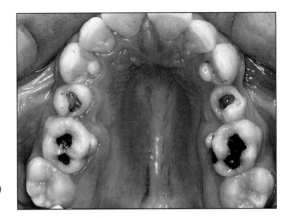

132 The high arched palate of the same patient (**130**, **131**) with Soto's syndrome.

Sturge–Weber syndrome (encephalofacial angiomatosis)

A neuroectodermal disorder in which angioma affects part of the face and usually extends into the occipital lobe of the brain, producing epilepsy and often hemiplegia and mental handicap (**133–135**). Radiography shows intracranial calcification of the angioma.

The haemangioma often appears to be limited to the area of distribution of one or more of the divisions of the trigeminal nerve. The affected area is somewhat swollen and hypertrophic.

The haemangioma may extend intraorally and be associated with hypertrophy of the affected jaw, macrodontia, and accelerated tooth eruption. Since the patients are often treated with phenytoin there may be gingival hyperplasia.

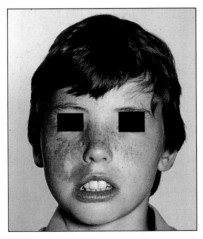

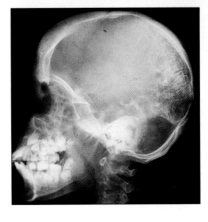

133 A 10-year-old boy with Sturge–Weber syndrome. There is an angioma affecting the maxillary division of the trigeminal nerve.

134 The palatal view of the boy in **133**. One side of the palate is slightly swollen and there are increased surface capillary markings. A primary canine has been shed from the unaffected side.

135 Intracranial calcification in Sturge–Weber syndrome.

Syphilis

Congenital syphilis is rare in developed countries. *Treponema pallidum*, the causal bacterium of this sexually transmitted disease, crosses the placenta only after the fifth month and can produce dental defects, typically Hutchinson's incisors (**136, 137**). These teeth have a barrel-shape, often with a notched incisal edge. Such dysplastic permanent incisors, along with neural deafness and interstitial keratitis, are combined in Hutchinson's triad. The molars may also be hypoplastic (Moon's molars or mulberry molars).

Other stigmata include scarring at the commissures (rhagades or Parrot's furrows), high-arched palate and a saddle-shaped nose. Frontal and parietal bossing (nodular focal osteoperiostitis of the frontal and parietal bones called Parrot's nodes) may be seen, and mental handicap is common.

136

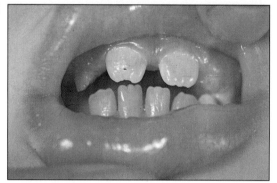

136 Hutchinson's incisors in congenital syphilis.

137

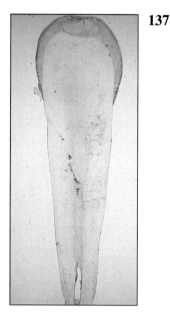

137 Hutchinson's incisor.

Torus mandibularis and torus palatinus

138

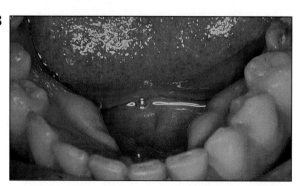

Mandibular tori are unilateral or bilateral bony lumps lingual to the lower premolars. They are of developmental origin and benign. Tori are common, especially in Mongoloid races (**138**).

Palatal tori are common bony lumps, typically in the midline vault of the palate. Palatal tori are most common in Mongoloid races and can sometimes be quite prominent. Again, they are benign.

138 Pronounced bilateral mandibular tori on the lingual side of the premolars in a Caucasian adolescent.

Trichorhinopharyngeal syndrome

This consists of cone-shaped epiphyses, sparse fine hair, bulbous nose with tented alae nasi and variable growth retardation (**139–142**). There may be midface hypoplasia, mild micrognathia, large outstanding ears and hypodontia.

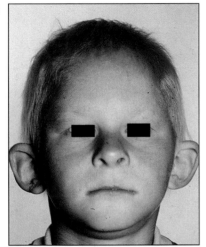

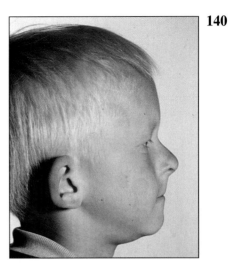

139, 140 A 5-year-old boy with somatic features characteristic of the trichorhinopharyngeal syndrome.

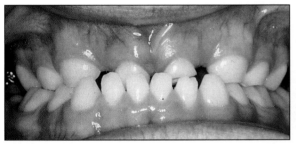

141 Hypodontia affecting the primary dentition in the patient in **139**. Both maxillary primary lateral incisors are missing. In the permanent dentition the maxillary lateral incisors and all the mandibular incisors failed to develop.

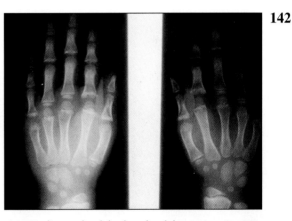

142 Radiograph of the hands of the patient in **139**. The left hand is clearer and shows cone-shaped epiphyses in all phalanges except the proximal phalanges of the middle and ring fingers and distal phalanx of the little finger. There is also a short fifth metacarpal and premature fusion of most epiphyses.

White sponge naevus (familial white folded gingivostomatosis)

White sponge naevus is a symptomless inconsequential autosomal dominant condition which manifests from infancy (**143**). The oral mucosa is thickened, folded, spongy and white or grey.

Oral lesions are bilateral; the vaginal or anal mucosa can also be affected.

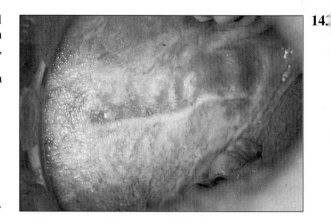

143

143 White sponge naevus.

Williams syndrome

The hypercalcaemia-supravalvular aortic stenosis syndrome is sometimes termed Williams syndrome. It comprises, in its rare complete form, infantile hypercalcaemia, characteristic so-called elfin facies, supravalvular aortic stenosis or other cardiovascular abnormalities and mental deficiency. Most such cases appear to be sporadic. Hypercalcaemia typically remits in infancy but leaves growth deficiency, osteosclerosis and craniostenosis. Despite the mental defect, these children may be sociable and talkative ('cocktail party manner').

Facial features, which become more striking with age, include a flat midface, depressed nasal bridge, anteverted nostrils, long philtrum, thick lips, wide inter-commissural distance and open mouth posture (**144, 145**). A high percentage of patients have blue eyes with a stellate iris pattern.

Hypodontia, microdontia, small slender roots, dens invaginatus, mild micrognathia, delayed mineralisation of teeth, and prominent and accessory labial fraenula may be present.

144

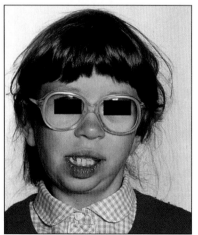

145

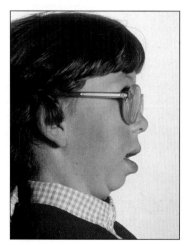

144 Frontal facial view illustrating the characteristic somatic features of Williams syndrome.

145 Lateral facial view illustrating the characteristic somatic features of Williams syndrome.

3. Disorders Affecting the Teeth

Abrasion

Abrasion is the wearing away of tooth substance by a habit such as toothbrushing. Brushing with a hard brush and coarse dentifrice may abrade the neck of the tooth (**146**). The gingiva recedes but is otherwise healthy. The cementum and dentine wear away but the harder enamel survives, resulting in a notch at the cervical margin. Abrasion is uncommon in children.

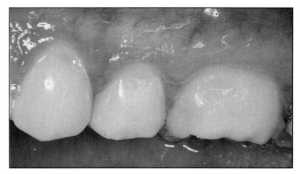

146

146 Toothbrush abrasion of the cervical regions of the maxillary premolars and first permanent molar in a teenager with poor toothbrushing technique.

Anomalies of eruption/tooth loss

Erupting permanent teeth may give rise to the appearance of a double row of teeth (**147**).

There is a wide variation in the eruption times of teeth. Early eruption is uncommon but may be seen, for example, in Soto's syndrome (**Table 1**). Delayed eruption is more common and typically affects only one or a few teeth, and is caused by physical obstruction to eruption (e.g. by tooth impaction). Delayed eruption of the whole dentition suggests a systemic cause: hypothyroidism is one example. The causes of early tooth loss are shown in **Table 2**.

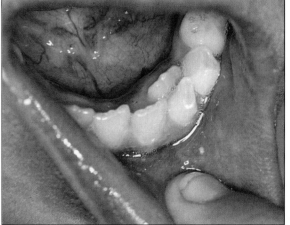

147

147 Permanent lateral incisor erupting lingual to a primary incisor. N.B. Gloves should now always be worn during patient care.

Table 1 Disorders associated with anomalies of tooth eruption in children.

NEONATAL TEETH

Ellis–van Creveld syndrome
Hallermann–Streiff syndrome
Pachyonychia congenita

PREMATURE ERUPTION

Precocious puberty
Hyperthyroidism
Hemifacial hypertrophy
Soto's syndrome
Sturge–Weber syndrome

DELAYED ERUPTION

Albright's hereditary osteodystrophy
Cleidocranial dysplasia
Down's syndrome
Hypothyroidism
Hypopituitarism
Gardner's syndrome
Goltz syndrome (focal dermal hypoplasia)
Incontinentia pigmenti

Table 2 Disorders causing loosening and early loss of teeth in children.

LOCAL CAUSES

Trauma
Periodontitis
Neoplasms (rarely)

SYSTEMIC CAUSES

Disorders with some immune deficit
    Down's syndrome
    Diabetes mellitus
    Leucopenia or leucocyte defects
    HIV disease
    Juvenile periodontitis
    Rapidly progressive periodontitis
    Papillon–Lefévre syndrome
Hypophosphatasia
Ehlers–Danlos syndrome (type VIII)

OTHERS

Acrodynia
Neoplasms
Eosinophilic granuloma
Hajdu–Cheney syndrome (acro-osteolysis syndrome)

Ankylosis

A primary molar may be retained, and in infraocclusion ('submerged') the permanent successor may be absent. There is then bony ankylosis and no evidence of a periodontal ligament (**148, 149**).

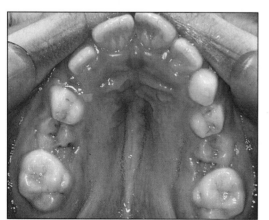

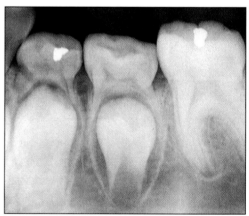

148 The maxillary second primary molars have undergone ankylosis to the underlying bone. Their occlusal surface is now considerably below the occlusal table and they are in danger of being covered by gingiva.

149 The mandibular second primary molar is ankylosed. There is little evidence of a periodontal ligament around either root.

Attrition

Attrition is the wearing away of tooth substance by mastication (**150**). It is uncommon in children but occurs where the diet is coarse or where there is a parafunctional habit such as bruxism (e.g. Rett's syndrome, *see* p. 40). The incisal edges and cusps wear with more loss of dentine than enamel, leading to a flat or hollowed surface but, unless attrition is rapid, the pulp is protected by secondary dentine formation.

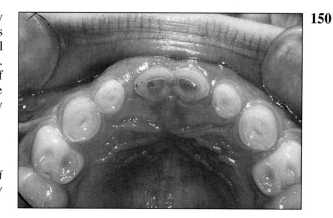

150

150 Marked attrition of the primary dentition as a result of an excessive grinding habit. The pulps of the maxillary central incisors are exposed.

Cusp of Carabelli

This is an anatomical variant—a palatal cusp on the upper first permanent molar (**151**).

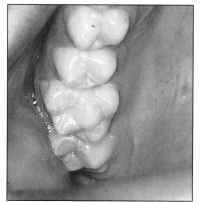

151

151 Prominent palatal cusp on a first maxillary permanent molar (cusp of Carabelli).

Dental bacterial plaque

Even after thorough toothbrushing, plaque often remains between the teeth unless they are flossed. Plaque is not especially obvious clinically, although teeth covered with it lack the lustre of clean teeth. Various chemicals can be used to disclose the plaque (**152**).

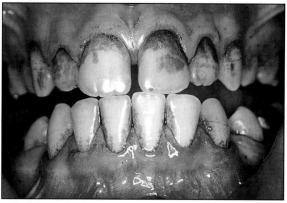

152

152 Plaque identified mainly around the gingival aspects of the teeth by utilising a disclosing solution containing vegetable dye.

Dental caries (decay)

Decalcification of tooth substance is caused by acids produced by sugar fermentation by the bacterial plaque that accumulates in stagnation areas, such as close to the gingival margin. Initially this produces an opaque whitish band. At this early stage, where there is no cavitation, the lesion is reversible if oral hygiene improves, the diet is changed (non-milk extrinsic sugars reduced or excluded) and topical fluoride is given (to aid remineralisation).

If unhalted, the carious enamel lesion breaks down to form a cavity and the dentine is invaded. The carious dentine is discoloured and this shows through the enamel (**153–155**). If untreated, caries almost inevitably progresses through the dentine to reach the dental pulp, which becomes inflamed. Such pulpitis causes pain and may result in pulp necrosis and dental abscess formation.

Change in dietary habits (particularly a reduction in total intake and frequency of intake of non-milk extrinsic sugars), topical fluoride treatment, and improved oral hygiene can arrest the progress of caries. Any change in local environment that makes the carious lesions self-cleansing—for example, loss of a tooth adjacent to an interproximal lesion, or fracture of cusps overlying a lesion—may cause arrest of the caries. Lesions then darken and become static.

In contrast, xerostomia significantly predisposes to caries. This may happen in children who have had radiotherapy to the tooth-bearing areas or salivary glands.

Rampant caries can affect mainly the upper incisors in a child using a sugared drink in a bottle to help sleep at night (**153**). Teeth do not erupt decayed, although with such a habit they can decay as they erupt.

153

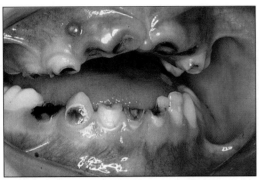

153 Extensive caries and sequelae in the primary dentition due to prolonged use of a night-comforter bottle containing a juice high in non-milk extrinsic sugars.

154

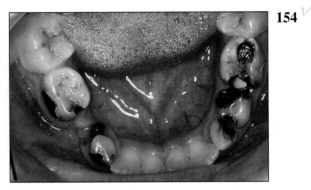

154 Extensive caries in a 9-year-old child due to excessive and frequent consumption of snack foods high in non-milk extrinsic sugars. The first permanent molars also had significant occlusal caries.

155

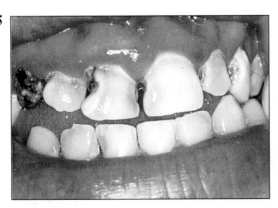

155 Advanced caries in the primary dentition.

Dilaceration

Trauma to a developing tooth may produce distortion and dilaceration (**156–158**)—a bend in either the root or the crown.

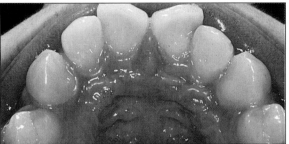

156 There is mesio-palatal rotation of the maxillary central permanent incisors (*see* **157**).

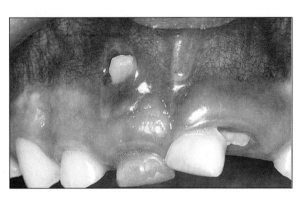

157 The corresponding radiograph reveals dilaceration of the middle third of the roots of these teeth. The patient's history revealed an episode of trauma to these teeth shortly after eruption.

158 There is a dilaceration of the root of the maxillary right central primary incisor so that the apex is visible in the buccal sulcus. The dilaceration occurred at the crown/root junction as a result of a fall at the age of 1 year. The apex has appeared in the buccal sulcus as a result of the permanent successor trying to erupt palatal to it.

Double teeth (connation)

Teeth joined together are often described by terms that are based on the suspected aetiology of the anomaly (**159–162**). For example, fusion is the term used to describe the union between the dentine and/or the enamel of two or more normally separate developing tooth germs. Gemination is the term used to describe the partial development of two teeth from a single tooth bud following incomplete division.

However, it is extremely difficult, if not impossible, to distinguish between fusion and gemination on clinical grounds. The number of normal teeth present is of little or no assistance as fusion may occur between a normal tooth and a supernumerary tooth, or between two supernumerary teeth. Alternatively, gemination could occur in a tooth germ adjacent to a congenitally absent tooth and this would be indistinguishable clinically from fusion. For these reasons a general descriptive term such as connation, which describes the appearance without suggesting the aetiology, is appropriate.

Connated ('developed' or 'born' together) teeth are more frequent in the primary dentition, and in the incisor or canine region. The condition may be bilaterally symmetrical and some families show a dominant trait of connated teeth.

159

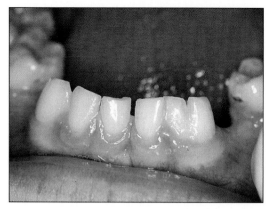

159 There is a connated tooth in the mandibular left primary canine region.

160

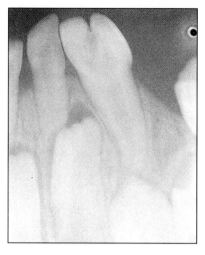

160 The periapical radiograph of the connated tooth in **161** shows a single root and a common pulp chamber in the crown.

161

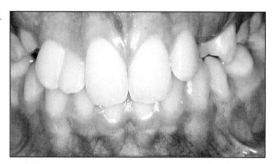

161 There is a connated tooth in the maxillary right permanent lateral incisor region.

162

162 The periapical radiograph of the connated tooth in **161** shows two separate dental elements joined only at the crowns, with no pulpal communication between the two elements.

Enamel cleft

Enamel clefts are often seen in the cervical region (**163**) and are probably due to a localised infolding of the ameloblast layer.

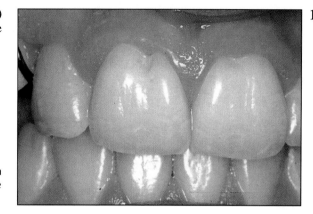

163 There is enamel clefting in the cervical region of both maxillary permanent central incisors, more obvious on the right central incisor.

Enamel hypoplasia

Tooth development can be disturbed by constitutional disturbances such as childhood febrile illnesses, cystic fibrosis and gastroenteritis, producing a linear pattern of defects corresponding to the site of amelogenesis at the time ('chronological' hypoplasia). Horizontal pits or grooves are usually seen in the incisal third of the crowns of permanent teeth. Intrauterine infections such as rubella, or metabolic disturbances, may cause hypoplasia of the primary dentition.

Infection of, or trauma to, a primary tooth may cause hypoplasia of the underlying permanent successor. Lower second premolars are not uncommonly deformed (Turner teeth) after an abscess on the predecessor primary molar. Enamel hypoplasia may also appear in the absence of any identifiable cause (**164–171**).

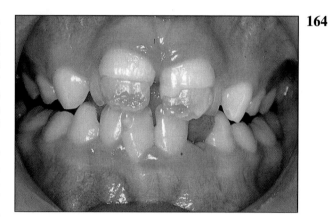

164 The enamel hypoplasia affecting the incisal half of the permanent incisors was a result of a well-documented episode of primary incisor trauma at the age of 9 months.

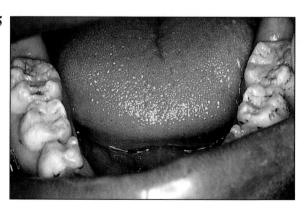

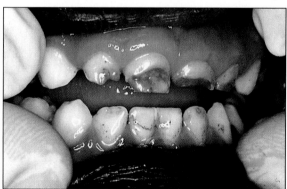

165, 166 The enamel hypoplasia seen on the incisors and primary molars was thought to be due to 1) maternal illness in the last trimester of pregnancy and 2) failure of the infant to thrive coupled with recurrent pneumonia in the first six months of life.

167

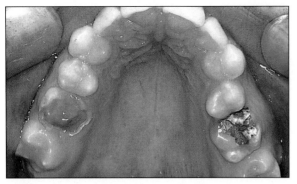

167 The enamel hypoplasia affecting the first permanent molars was thought to be due to a prolonged and difficult labour complicated by pre-eclamptic toxaemia.

168

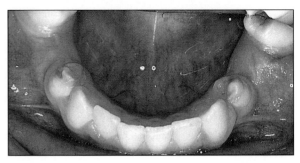

168 Both mandibular first permanent premolars are hypoplastic. The predecessor first primary molars had both had periapical abscesses.

169

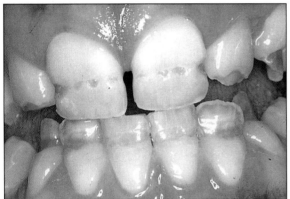

169 The chronological hypoplasia affecting the maxillary and mandibular permanent incisors was probably due to severe measles during the second year of life.

170

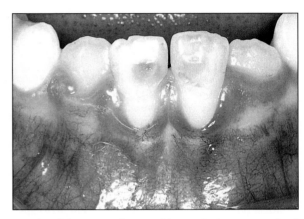

170 A milder case of enamel hypoplasia as a result of trauma to the primary predecessor. Both mandibular permanent central incisors have localised areas of staining and pitting.

171

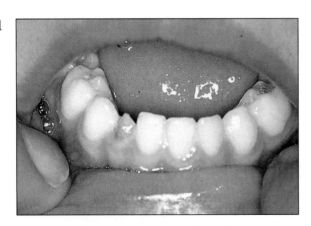

171 Isolated enamel hypoplasia in a permanent lateral incisor (Turner tooth). N.B. Gloves should now always be worn during patient care.

Erosion

Erosion is the loss of tooth substance caused by acids. Citrus fruits, carbonated beverages or recurrent vomiting may produce such lesions, which are more common in adolescents than younger children (**172–175**).

Repeated gastric regurgitation over a prolonged period may cause erosion, mainly of the palatal surfaces of the upper teeth. This is seen especially in bulimia nervosa.

Other features of bulimia include enlargement of salivary glands—sialosis(mainly parotids); palatal petechiae; possible conjunctival suffusion and oesophageal tears (caused by retching); and Russell's sign—abrasions on the back of the hand or fingers caused by using the fingers to induce vomiting.

172
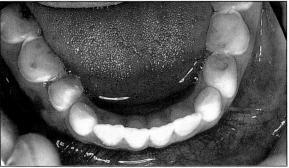

172 Marked erosion of the occlusal surface of the mandibular second primary molars and first permanent molars as a result of frequent intakes of lime and lemon juice cordial.

173
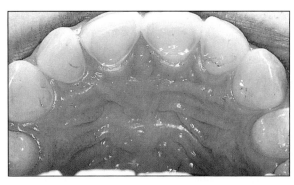

173 Palatal erosion of the maxillary permanent canines and incisors in a cola drink addict.

174
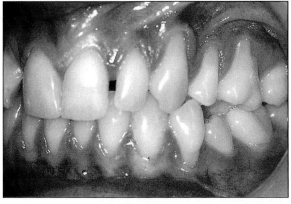

175
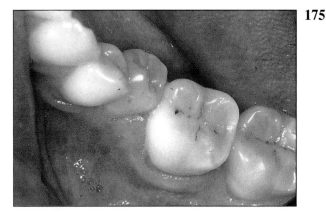

174, 175 Erosion of both the occlusal and labial enamel in an adolescent with bulimia nervosa. In addition, there is marked recession of labial gingiva due to an incorrect brushing technique.

Eruption cyst

The eruption cyst is a type of dentigerous cyst, i.e. it surrounds the crown of the tooth. This cyst often presents clinically as a smooth, rounded swelling with a bluish appearance if there is no overlying bone. Eruption cysts most often involve the primary teeth and permanent molars (i.e. teeth with no predecessors) (**176**).

Eruption cysts often break down spontaneously as the tooth erupts.

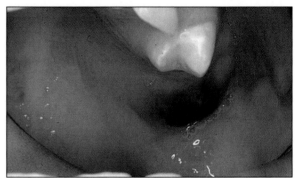

176

176 An eruption cyst in the maxillary right quadrant heralding the imminent eruption of the second permanent molar tooth. The permanent second premolar and first molar have been extracted because of gross caries.

External resorption

External resorption (**177**) is usually either a response to trauma of the periodontal ligament, or secondary to pulpal necrosis. It is initiated in the periodontium and progresses from the external surface, eventually to involve the pulp.

177

177 External inflammatory resorption affecting most of the root of a replanted maxillary permanent central incisor. The 'tram lines' of the root canal are still evident despite the 'moth-eaten' appearance of the root. This fact helps to distinguish external inflammatory resorption from internal inflammatory resorption, which is initiated from within the root canal.

Extrinsic staining

Extrinsic staining of the teeth can be of various colours and is more likely to appear where oral hygiene is poor (**178–180**). Smoking, coloured foods and beverages (spices, tea and coffee), and medicines such as chlorhexidine, iron, or minocycline may be implicated (**Table 3**).

Orange stain is believed to be caused by chromogenic bacteria. Brown stain is concentrated mainly where plaque accumulates, such as between the teeth, close to the gingival margins and in pits and fissures. It is usually due to food and beverages but can be caused by stannous fluoride toothpaste or chlorhexidine. Black stain is of unknown aetiology, often seen in clean mouths, and is unusual in that it seems, by an unknown mechanism, to be associated with caries resistance. Green stain is most common in children with poor oral hygiene and may result from breakdown of blood pigment after gingival haemorrhage, or from chromogenic bacteria.

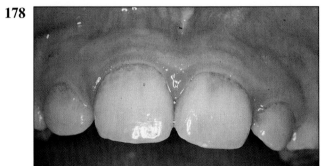

178 Orange stain.

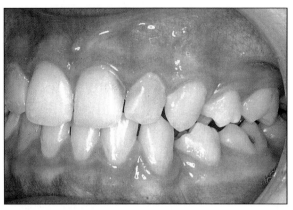

179 Green stain affecting the maxillary central and lateral permanent incisors as a result of poor oral hygiene.

Table 3 Causes of discolouration of teeth in children.

EXTRINSIC

Poor oral hygiene
Smoking
Beverages/food
Drugs, e.g. iron, chlorhexidine, minocycline
Stains (orange, green, brown, black)

INTRINSIC

Trauma
Caries
Restorative materials, e.g. amalgam
Pink spot (internal resorption)
Tetracyclines
Fluorosis
Dentinogenesis imperfecta
Amelogenesis imperfecta
Porphyria
Kernicterus (severe neonatal jaundice)

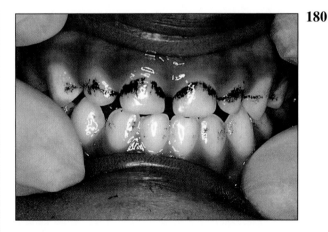

180 Black extrinsic stain affecting the primary dentition in an Ethiopian child who had a high intake of spicy foods and tea.

Hyperdontia

Additional teeth (**181–190**) can closely resemble the normal dentition (supplemental teeth) or be a simple conical shape (supernumerary teeth). In the midline, a supernumerary tooth is termed a mesiodens and may be inverted.

Unerupted supernumerary teeth often impede normal tooth eruption or, more rarely, are the site of cyst formation as a cause of external resorption. Erupted supernumerary teeth can cause a malocclusion and may then predispose to caries or periodontal disease.

Occasionally, supernumerary teeth are a manifestation of a systemic disorder such as cleidocranial dysplasia (*see* p. 14) or Gardner's syndrome (desmoid tumours, osteomas and colonic polyps) (**Table 4**).

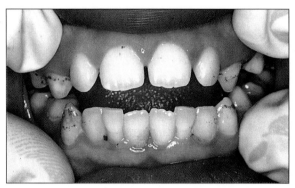

181 Retained mandibular primary lateral incisors between central and lateral permanent incisors.

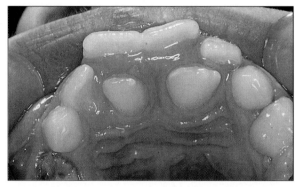

182 Supplemental maxillary permanent lateral incisors have erupted palatal to the normal incisors.

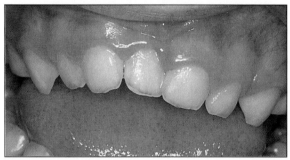

183 A supplemental primary central incisor has erupted in the midline between the normal primary central incisors.

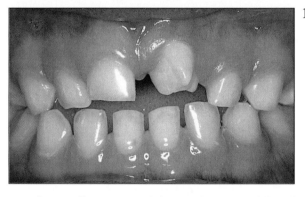

184 The maxillary primary left central incisor exfoliated prematurely due to the eruption of a supernumerary element with a labially positioned 'talon' cusp.

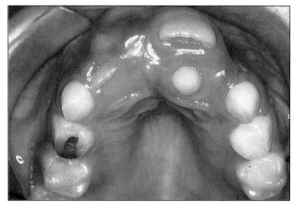

185 There is an erupted supernumary tooth palatal to the left maxillary central incisor. The right maxillary permanent central incisor is just visible high in the labial sulcus.

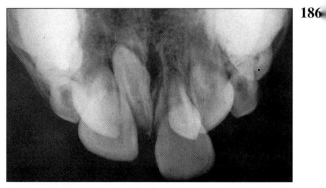

186 The radiograph of **185** shows an inverted mesiodens which has impeded the eruption of the right maxillary permanent central incisor. The erupted left palatal supernumerary is also visible.

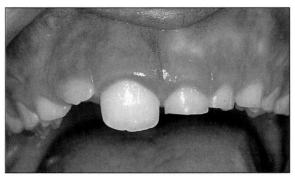

187 There is failure of eruption of the maxillary left permanent central incisor, due to a supernumerary tooth.

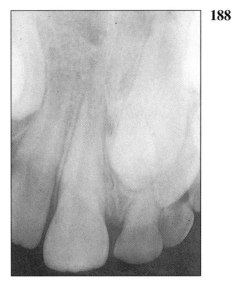

188 Radiography of the patient in **187** shows a mesiodens lying palatal to the crown of the unerupted tooth.

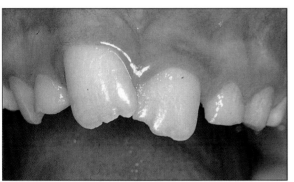

189 Both maxillary permanent central incisors have erupted but the right central incisor is not in alignment.

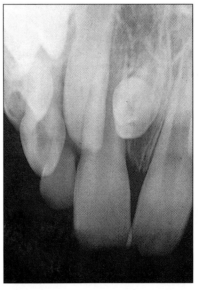

190 The radiograph from **189** shows a palatally positioned mesiodens which has pushed the root and apex of the right central incisor distally.

Table 4 Disorders associated with anomalies of tooth number.

HYPODONTIA

Albright's hereditary osteodystrophy
Cretinism
Down's syndrome
Ectodermal dysplasia
Goltz's syndrome (focal dermal hypoplasia)
Hallermann–Streiff's syndrome
Incontinentia pigmenti
Oral-facial digital syndromes
Cleft lip and palate

SUPERNUMERARY TEETH

Cleidocranial dysplasia
Gardner's syndrome
Hallermann–Streiff's syndrome
Cleft lip and palate

Hyperplastic pulpitis (pulp polyp)

Only when the coronal pulp is widely exposed and there is a very good blood supply does the pulp survive trauma or carious infection. This situation can, however, occur in primary teeth or occasionally in first permanent molars and the pulp then becomes hyperplastic and epithelialised, producing a polyp (**191**).

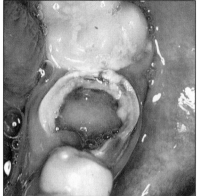

191

191 Pulp polyp in a mandibular first molar.

Hypodontia

Teeth may appear missing because they are unerupted. This may be because they are impacted and thus fail to erupt or, more rarely, eruption is delayed due to systemic disease, such as cretinism or Down's syndrome.

Cytotoxic drugs and radiotherapy may also cause retarded eruption of teeth (**195**).

Isolated hypodontia (**192–200**) is fairly common, may have a genetic basis, and affects mainly the permanent dentition, particularly third molars, second premolars or upper lateral incisors. Hypodontia is often associated with microdontia and is often bilaterally symmetrical. The primary tooth is then commonly retained. Usually this is of little consequence, but the retained tooth may fail to keep its occlusal relationship, particularly in lower primary molars (infraocclusion or submergence).

Hypodontia is a feature of local disorders such as cleft palate, and of many systemic disorders. In some, the teeth are present but fail to erupt; in others, such as ectodermal dysplasia, or incontinentia pigmenti, they are truly missing (**Table 4**). Rarely, all teeth are absent (anodontia).

192

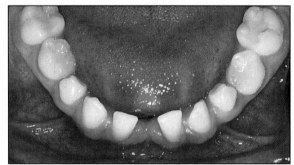

192 Hypodontia affecting the maxillary and mandibular arches in a 15-year-old male.

193, 194 Teeth 65, 75, 85 are retained and teeth 16, 15, 14, 12, 24, 25, 26, 37, 35, 31, 41, 45, 47 are missing. The maxillary central incisors have been traumatised and subsequently repaired with composite resin. There was no associated medical condition and no previous family history of hypodontia.

193

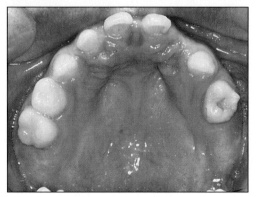

19

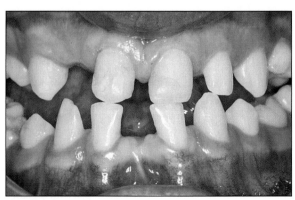

195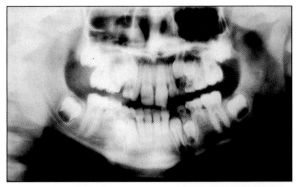

195 The radiograph shows failure of development of all permanent second premolars in a patient who had received chemotherapy between the ages of 2–2$^1/_2$ years for the treatment of Wilm's tumour.

196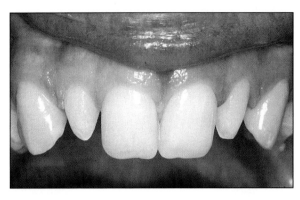

196 Bilateral conical 'peg-shaped' permanent lateral incisors. There is often a family history of the same, or of a peg-shaped lateral incisor on one side and absence on the contralateral side or of a bilaterally absent lateral incisors.

197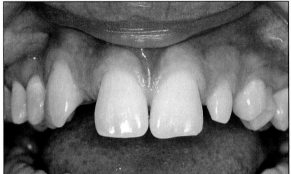

197 A peg-shaped permanent lateral incisor in the maxillary left quadrant, with congenital absence of the maxillary right lateral incisor.

198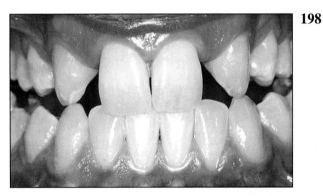

198 Bilateral congenital absence of both maxillary permanent lateral incisors.

199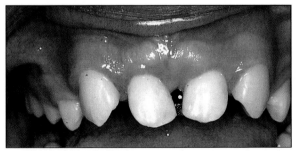

199 Traumatic hypodontia. Both maxillary permanent central incisors were lost at an earlier age due to trauma. The lateral incisors have drifted mesially.

200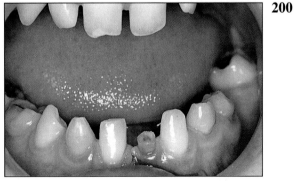

200 Hypodontia with retained non-vital primary tooth.

Impacted teeth

Lower third molars are the most common teeth to impact, that is, fail to erupt fully because of insufficient space. Canines and second premolars also commonly impact.

Impacted teeth may be asymptomatic but occasionally cause pain, usually from pericoronitis or caries, or are the site of dentigerous cyst formation (**201–203**).

201

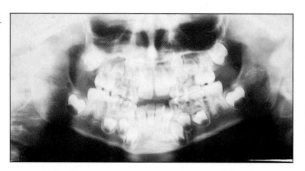

201 The left maxillary first permanent molar has not erupted fully into the arch but has impacted into the distal surface of the second primary molar. This is an occasional finding with no obvious cause.

202

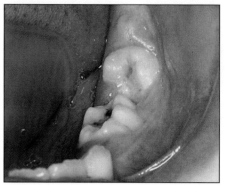

202 The mandibular first permanent molar has erupted mesially to impact against the second primary molar. Such impactions are commoner in mandibular third molars. There was no obvious cause for the impaction in this case.

203

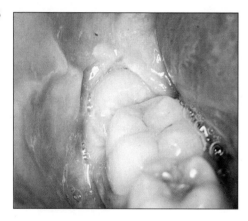

203 Impacted mandibular third molar (wisdom tooth).

Internal resorption (pink spot)

In this, dentine is spontaneously resorbed from within (204–206). The pulp is eventually exposed.

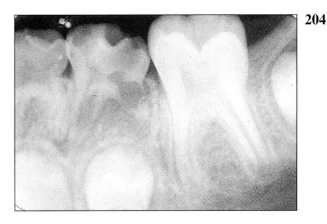

204

204 There is internal resorption affecting both the roots of the mandibular second primary molar. The architecture of the root canal is lost and there is ballooning of the canal as successive amounts of dentine are replaced with inflammatory and granulation tissue. The stimulus for internal resorption is from the necrotic products of pulpal necrosis.

205

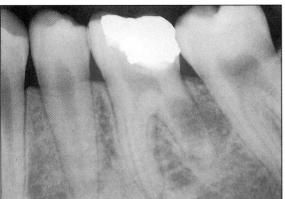

205 There is internal resorption affecting the distal root of the mandibular first permanent molar.

206

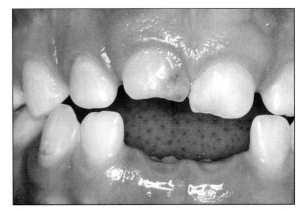

206 Internal resorption in a primary maxillary right central incisor occurring naturally in a tooth about to be exfoliated. The pink hue produced by granulation tissue within the crown is visible.

Intrinsic staining

Whitish flecks in the enamel are not uncommon and are often idiopathic (**207**). Mottling of the enamel may be seen where the fluoride in drinking water exceeds about 2 ppm or where excess fluoride is taken via other sources. Mottling in mild fluorosis is usually seen as white flecks or patches. Severe fluorosis causes brown and white mottling and pitting of the entire enamel. This can be difficult clinically to differentiate from amelogenesis imperfecta. The mottling is often severe enough to require cosmetic treatment of the upper anterior teeth (**208–210**).

Haemolytic disease of the newborn (icterus gravis neonatorum) (**211**) is now rare and more infants survive with hyperbilirubinaemia due to other causes. Jaundice in either case may cause enamel hypoplasia, usually in the primary dentition, which may have a greenish colour (**212**). Congenital erythropoietic porphyria is a rare cause of yellow to brown-red tooth discolouration.

Tetracyclines are a relatively common cause of tooth staining (**54, 213–216**). Tetracyclines are taken up by developing teeth and by bone, and, if given to pregnant or nursing mothers or to children under the age of 8 years, the tooth crowns become discoloured.

Tetracycline staining is most obvious in light-exposed anterior teeth, initially being yellow but darkening with time. Staining of the permanent dentition—yellow and brown bands of staining—is most obvious at the necks of the teeth where the thinner enamel allows the colour of the stained dentine to show through. Staining is greater the larger the dose of tetracycline, and is least with oxytetracycline. Affected teeth may fluoresce bright yellow under ultraviolet light, and this helps to distinguish tetracycline staining from dentinogenesis imperfecta. Fluorescence is also seen in undecalcified sections viewed under ultraviolet light.

In older children most tooth crowns have formed and tetracycline staining then affects only the roots.

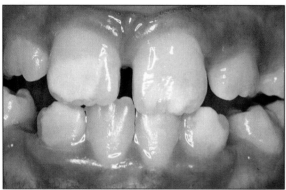

207 Idiopathic white patches affecting the permanent maxillary central and mandibular lateral incisors.

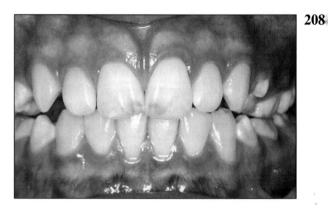

208 Mild fluorosis. There are diffuse white opacities affecting all the permanent teeth. In addition, there is brown staining of the maxillary central incisors and both maxillary and mandibular first permanent molars. This patient had lived from birth to the age of 7 years in Tanzania where there was a naturally fluoridated water supply.

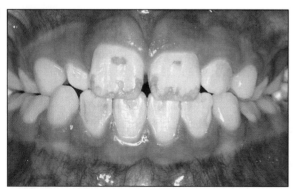

209 A more severe case of fluorosis than **208**. The brown staining on the maxillary incisors is more extensive and darker in colour. This patient had a well-documented history of eating fluoridated toothpaste.

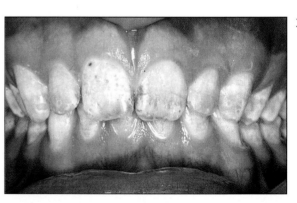

210 Severe fluorosis with pitting of the enamel as well as white and brown mottling. This patient had been brought up in the Far East where there was not only a naturally fluoridated water supply but also fluoride supplements in the form of tablets had been taken.

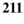

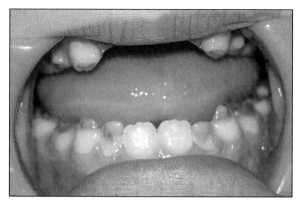

211 Kernicterus showing pigmented enamel hypoplasia of the primary teeth.

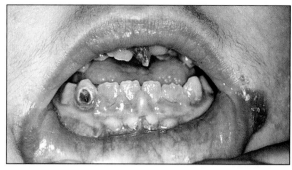

212 Bile pigment staining of teeth in congenital liver disease. There is also oral neglect with caries, and gingival hyperplasia produced by cyclosporin therapy after liver transplantation.

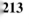

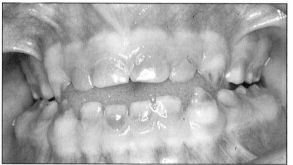

213 Tetracycline staining of the primary dentition as a result of maternal treatment with tetracycline during pregnancy.

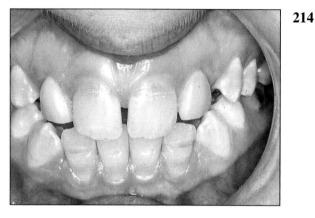

214 Grey tetracycline staining of the permanent dentition with banding in the cervical regions. In addition, there is hypoplasia of the mandibular incisors affecting the middle third of the crowns. (The maxillary lateral incisors have been veneered.)

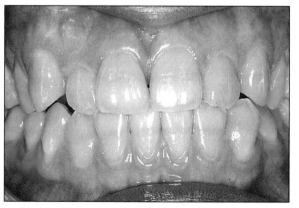

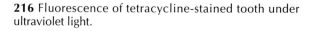

215 Intense yellow tetracycline staining of the permanent dentition. Banding is more evident in the mandibular incisors.

216 Fluorescence of tetracycline-stained tooth under ultraviolet light.

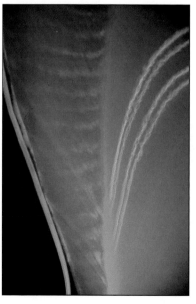

Macrodontia

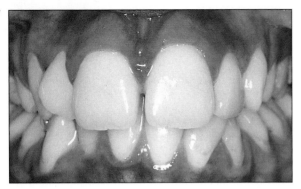

217

In true generalised macrodontia (**217**) all the teeth are larger than normal. In hemihypertrophy of the face the teeth of the involved side may be larger than the unaffected side.

217 True generalised macrodontia. Both maxillary permanent central incisors were 12 mm in diameter.

Malocclusion

Textbooks of orthodontics give full details of this subject (**218–222**).

Mandibular retrusion is common but only rarely results in a typical 'bird face'.

Maxillary protrusion is also common and this type of malocclusion is termed a class II malocclusion.

Mandibular protrusion (Class III malocclusion) is uncommon but typically associated with the Hapsburg chin of a prognathic mandible. In mandibular protrusion, the teeth often show reverse overjet with the upper incisors occluding lingual to the lowers.

In anterior open bite, the posterior teeth are in occlusion but the incisors fail to meet. Anterior open bites may be caused not only by increased height of the lower face but occasionally by tongue posture, trauma or thumb-sucking.

Crowding of teeth is very common, particularly in the canine, second premolar, and lower incisor regions. The permanent canines normally erupt slightly later than the premolars and lateral incisors and, if there is lack of space in the dental arch (dentoalveolar disproportion), they are crowded out of the dental arch. Second premolars and third molars are the other teeth that may suffer this fate. Any of these teeth, especially lower third molars, may impact. The lower incisors are frequently crowded and malaligned (imbricated).

218

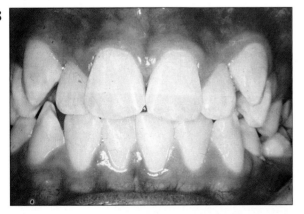

218 Crowding. There is insufficient space for the maxillary permanent canine teeth which have erupted buccal to the arch, resulting in them becoming more prominent.

219

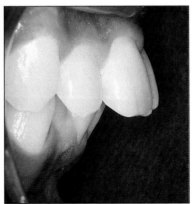

219 Class II malocclusion type I. The maxillary permanent central incisors are prominent, and, with the posterior teeth in occlusion the lips will not be able to cover the anterior teeth whilst at rest. The overjet in this case was 11 mm.

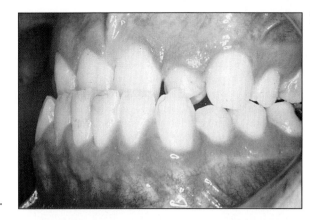

220 Class III malocclusion.

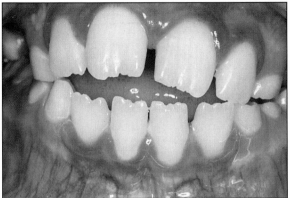

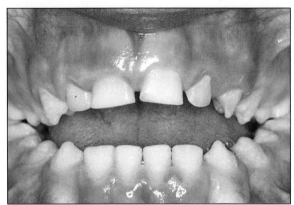

221, 222 Anterior open bite. The posterior teeth are in occlusion but the incisors fail to meet.

Materia alba

In extreme examples of poor oral hygiene, the teeth are covered with a soft white cheesy deposit of debris from food, effete epithelial cells, and dental plaque (**223**). Neglected handicapped chldren are the most frequently seen with this problem: gingivitis usually follows, as shown here.

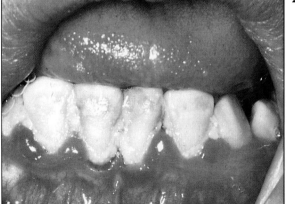

223 Materia alba covering the mandibular anterior teeth with associated gingivitis.

Odontomes

Odontomes are a group of non-neoplastic, developmental anomalies or malformations derived from dental formative tissues. They contain fully formed enamel and dentine and can be considered as dental hamartomas.

The complex odontome (**224**) consists of a mass of irregularly arranged dental tissue in which enamel, dentine, cementum and pulpal tissue are represented. The compound odontome comprises numerous discrete tooth-like structures, which may not resemble teeth of the normal dentition but in which enamel, dentine, cementum and pulp are arranged as in a normal tooth.

Invagination of enamel and dentine (dilated odontome; dens in dente; dens invaginatus) (**225**) may also dilate the affected tooth. Ameloblasts invaginate during development to form a pouch of enamel such that a radiograph shows what resembles a tooth within a tooth. This odontome is prone to caries development in the abnormal pouch. Pulpitis may follow.

A small occlusal nodule (**226**) (evaginated odontome; dens evaginatus) may be seen, especially in mongoloid races. Since the nodule contains a pulp horn, pulpitis is not uncommon when there is attrition.

224

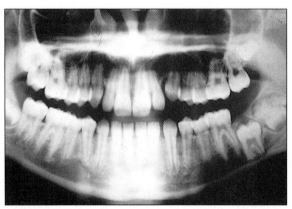

224 A complex odontome in the left mandibular angle arising from a developing third permanent molar. The patient had received chemotherapy from 8–10$^1/_2$ years of age, for acute lymphoblastic leukaemia.

225

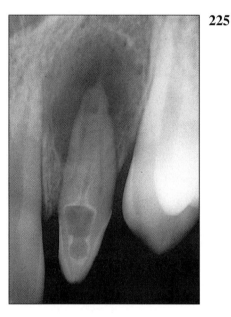

225 An invaginated odontome of the maxillary permanent left lateral incisor. Pulpal infection has resulted in a large periapical abscess.

226

226 Dens evaginatus in the second premolar.

Periapical abscess (dental abscess, odontogenic abscess) and cyst

An abscess is often a sequel of pulpitis caused by dental caries but may arise in relation to any non-vital tooth (e.g. subsequent to trauma) (227–231). A mixed bacterial flora is implicated, although the role of anaerobes such as fusobacteria and bacteroides species is increasingly recognised. Pain and facial swelling are characteristic. Most dental abscesses produce an intraoral swelling, typically on the labial or buccal gingiva. However, abscesses on maxillary lateral incisors and those arising from the palatal roots of the first molar may present palatally. Occasionally, abscesses—especially those of lower incisors or molars—discharge extraorally.

Once the abscess discharges beyond the periosteum, the acute inflammation, pain and swelling resolve and a chronic abscess develops, discharging from a sinus—usually buccally.

Extraction, or endodontic therapy of the affected tooth, removes the source of infection.

A granuloma may arise at the apex of a non-vital tooth and may occasionally develop into a cyst from proliferation of epithelial rests in the area (cell rests of Malassez). Many periapical cysts (229, 230) involve upper lateral incisors since these not infrequently become carious and the pulp can be involved relatively rapidly. A periapical cyst may well be asymptomatic and is often a chance radiographic finding. It may present as a swelling (usually in the labial sulcus) or may become infected and present as an abscess.

A small periapical cyst may remain attached to, and be extracted with, the causal root or tooth, or resolve with endodontic therapy.

A periapical cyst left *in situ* after the causal root or tooth is removed may continue to expand, and is termed a residual cyst. This is almost invariably unilocular but may expand to an appreciable size. It may be asymptomatic, may be detected as a swelling (231), a chance radiographic finding, or it may become infected and present as an abscess or, very rarely, as a pathological fracture.

Most odontogenic cysts are periapical.

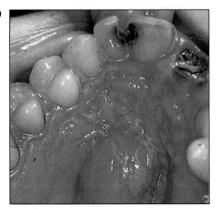

227 Acute periapical abscess arising from a traumatised necrotic maxillary primary central incisor.

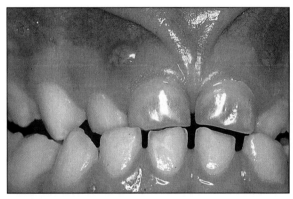

228 Both maxillary primary incisors are non-vital and have periapical infection pointing buccally.

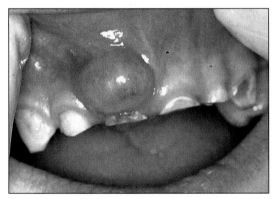

229 Acute periapical abscess arising from a carious maxillary permanent incisor.

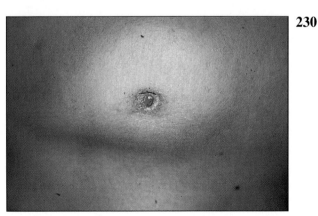

230 Periapical abscess from a lower permanent incisor, discharging on to skin of the chin.

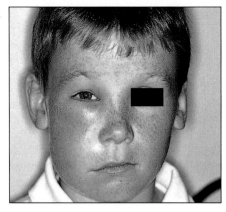

231 Facial swelling associated with a periapical abscess.

Prominent tubercles or cusps

Teeth are occasionally malformed with a large palatal cusp, sometimes to the extent that they have a talon cusp configuration (**232–234**).

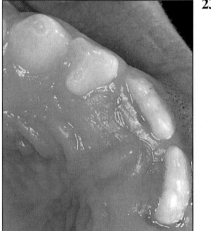

232 A talon cusp of the maxillary right lateral primary incisor. Such prominent cusps in either the primary or the permanent dentitions may interfere with occlusion and thus necessitate treatment.

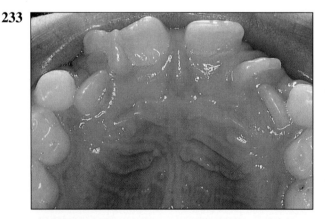

233 There is a large connated tooth in the maxillary right permanent central incisor position which also has a prominent palatal (talon) cusp. On the other side of the arch there is a supplemental lateral incisor. In this case the connated tooth has probably arisen due to fusion between the normal central incisor and a supplemental element.

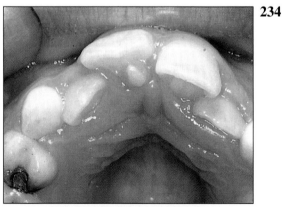

234 A prominent palatal cusp on the cingulum area of the maxillary permanent right central incisor.

Taurodontism

Taurodontism is the term applied to teeth that clinically look normal but, on a radiograph (**235**), resemble those of ungulates (hence the Latin origin, *taurus*, a bull). The crown is long, the roots short. Taurodont teeth lack a pronounced constriction at the neck of the tooth and are parallel-sided. The floor of the pulp chamber is lower than normal and the pulp appears extremely large. Taurodontism usually affects permanent molars, especially the lower second molar, sometimes only one in the arch, but may affect teeth in the primary dentition.

Taurodontism is usually a simple trait but may rarely be associated with a systemic disorder such as Klinefelter's syndrome, tricho-dento-osseous syndrome, oral-facial-digital syndrome, or ectodermal dysplasia.

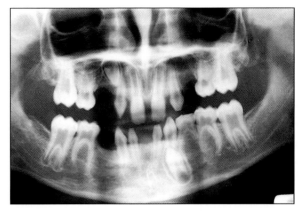

235

235 Taurodontism of the maxillary and mandibular first permanent molars.

Transposition

A transposition is when the normal positions of two teeth are reversed (**236**).

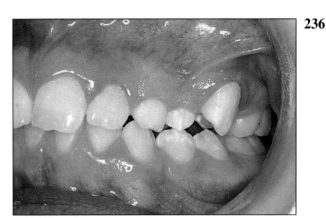

236

236 Transposition: the maxillary permanent left canine has erupted distal and buccal to the first premolar.

Trauma

While any tooth can be traumatised it is mainly the maxillary incisors, particularly in boys, that are damaged. The damage to a crown can involve the enamel alone, or can extend to involve the dentine or even pulp (**237**). The pulps of affected teeth may become necrotic after trauma (and then darken with time), or the tooth may be subluxed or lost completely. Ultimately, a periapical abscess may result.

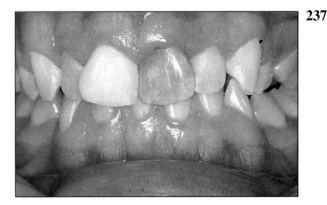

237

237 The maxillary permanent left central incisor is non-vital and discoloured as a result of trauma some years previously. Products of blood breakdown and pulpal necrosis have passed into the dentinal tubules to give the dark blue-grey appearance.

4. Acquired Gingival and Periodontal Diseases

Acute necrotising gingivitis (Vincent's disease)

Chiefly affecting young adults, acute necrotising gingivitis (acute necrotising ulcerative gingivitis, AUG, ANG, ANUG) (238, 239) is associated with proliferation of *Borrelia vincentii*, fusiform bacilli and other anaerobes. Painful ulceration of the interdental papillae is the typical feature of this condition. Painful gingival papillary ulceration occasionally spreads from the papillae to the gingival margins (*see also* cancrum oris, p. 72). There is often accompanying sialorrhoea, halitosis, and a pronounced tendency to gingival bleeding. Acute necrotising gingivitis is predisposed by respiratory infections, poor oral hygiene, smoking and immune defects. HIV infection is now a recognised predisposing factor in some patients.

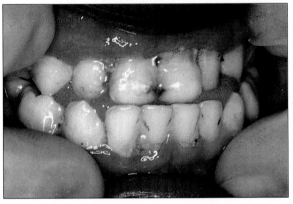

238 Acute necrotising gingivitis affecting the maxillary and mandibular anterior regions in a 6-year-old child. Oral hygiene and nutrient intake were poor.

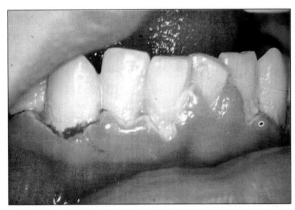

239 Acute necrotising gingivitis showing papillary and marginal gingival ulceration.

Acute pericoronitis

In acute pericoronitis (240, 241) inflammation of the operculum over an erupting or impacted tooth is common. The lower third molar is the site most commonly affected, but it is occasionally seen in relation to second molars. Patients complain of pain, trismus, swelling and halitosis. There may be fever and regional lymphadenitis, the operculum is swollen, red and often ulcerated and there may be halitosis.

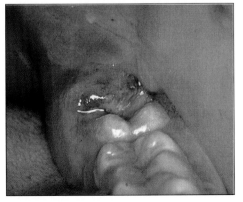

240 Acute pericoronitis associated with a partially erupted mandibular permanent molar.

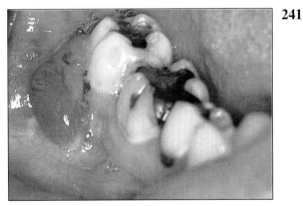

241 Migratory abscess of the buccal sulcus—a rare sequel of acute pericoronitis.

Cancrum oris (noma)

Although usually a trivial illness in healthy children, ANG in malnourished, debilitated, or severely immunocompromised patients may extend onto the oral mucosa and skin with gangrenous necrosis (cancrum oris, noma) (**242**). Though strictly a mucosal disorder, it typically originates at the gingiva. Anaerobes, particularly bacteroides species, have been implicated, and the condition is especially seen in malnourished patients from the developing world or war zones. Gangrenous stomatitis has also been reported in HIV disease.

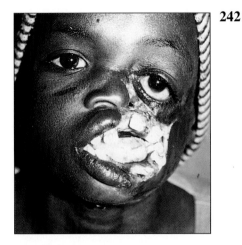

242

242 Cancrum oris in an African child.

Chronic hyperplastic gingivitis

Gingivitis may be hyperplastic (**243–245, Table 5**), especially where there is mechanical irritation, or mouth-breathing, or sometimes with the use of some drugs (*see* below).

243

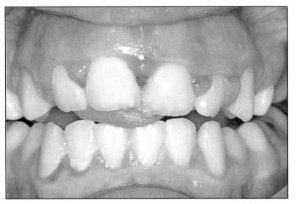

244

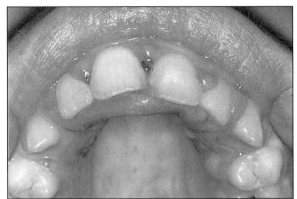

243, 244 Chronic hyperplastic gingivitis affecting the maxillary labial and palatal gingivae, and after orthodontic removable appliance treatment to retract teeth in the upper labial segment.

245

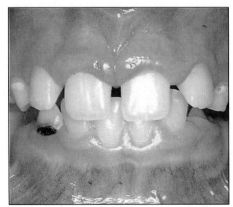

245 Chronic hyperplastic gingivitis in a mouth-breather.

Table 5 Main causes of gingival swelling in childhood.

	Generalised	Localised
Local	Chronic gingivitis Hyperplastic gingivitis due to mouth-breathing	Abscesses Cysts Warts Pyogenic granuloma Neoplasms (rarely)
Systemic	Hereditary gingival fibromatosis and associated syndromes Drugs: Phenytoin Cyclosporin Nifedipine Diltiazem Felodipine Sarcoidosis Crohn's disease Leukaemia Scurvy Mucopolysaccharidoses Mucolipidosis Juvenile hyaline fibromatosis	Sarcoidosis Orofacial granulomatosis Crohn's disease Neoplasms (rarely)

Chronic marginal gingivitis

Most of the adult population have a degree of gingivitis, which commences in childhood. Chronic marginal gingivitis (**246, 247**) is caused by the accumulation of dental plaque on the tooth close to the gingiva. If plaque is not removed it calcifies to become calculus and this aggravates the condition by facilitating plaque accumulation.

Inflammation of the margins of the gingiva is painless, and often the only features are gingival bleeding on eating or brushing, and possibly some halitosis. There may be gingival erythema, swelling, and bleeding on examination. If left uncorrected, gingivitis may slowly and painlessly progress to periodontitis and ultimately to tooth loss.

246

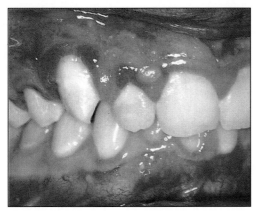

246 Chronic marginal gingivitis, especially of the maxillary gingiva.

247

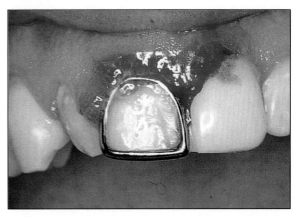

247 Marginal gingivitis closely related to a restoration (a basket crown—now outdated).

Dental calculus

248

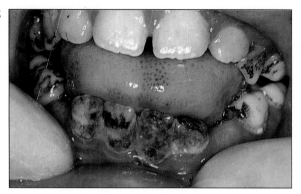

If plaque is not removed it readily calcifies to produce calculus (tartar) (**248**) on the teeth, especially in sites close to salivary duct orifices, e.g. lingual to the lower incisors and buccal to the upper molars.

Calculus cannot be removed by toothbrushing, and may be associated with periodontal disease.

248 Calculus, covering the mandibular incisors in a 10-year-old child, is itself covered by plaque and significant extrinsic stain (an extreme example).

Drug-induced gingival hyperplasia

The anticonvulsant phenytoin is the drug which traditionally can produce gingival hyperplasia (**249–251, Table 5**). Poor oral hygiene exacerbates the hyperplasia, which appears interdentally 2–3 months after treatment is started. The gingival papillae enlarge to a variable extent, with relatively little tendency to bleed, and may even cover the tooth crowns.

Cyclosporin is a commonly used immunosuppressive drug that can cause gingival hyperplasia closely resembling that induced by phenytoin. It is seen mainly anteriorly and labially and is exacerbated by concurrent administration of nifedipine.

Nifedipine is a calcium channel blocker occasionally used as an antihypertensive in children; it can produce gingival hyperplasia, similar to that induced by phenytoin. Some other antihypertensives can cause gingival hyperplasia.

All types of drug-induced gingival hyperplasia may also be associated with hirsutism.

249

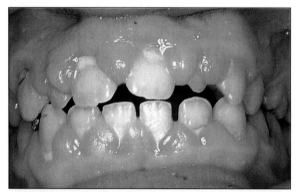

250

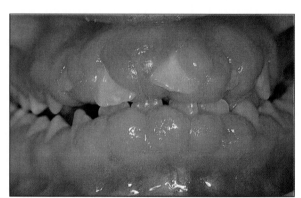

251

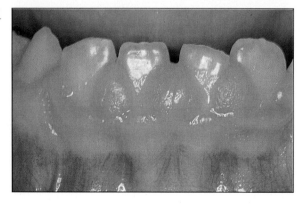

249, 250 Phenytoin-induced gingival hyperplasia.

251 Cyclosporin-induced gingival hyperplasia in a 9-year-old child. The drug had been taken regularly for 2 years following a heart transplant.

Fibroepithelial polyps and pyogenic granulomas

Fibroepithelial polyps (fibrous lump) (**252**) are common in the mouth, but are seen mainly in adults. They appear to be purely reparative in nature.

The variable inflammatory changes account for the different clinical presentations of fibrous lumps from red, shiny and soft lumps to those which are pale, stippled and firm. Commonly, they are round, pedunculated swellings arising from the marginal or papillary gingiva (epulides), and sometimes adjacent to sites of irritation (e.g. a carious cavity). They are usually painless. They may reach quite a large size, but the prognosis is good.

The true fibroma, a benign neoplasm of fibroblastic origin, is rare in the oral cavity, and many lesions called fibromas in the past were probably fibroepithelial polyps.

Pyogenic granuloma, which commonly affects the gingiva, the lip or the tongue (**253, 254**), is an exaggerated response to minor trauma. It tends to manifest in the form of soft, fleshy, rough-surfaced, vascular lesions that bleed readily. Most pyogenic granulomas are seen in the maxilla, anteriorly. The gingiva is the most common site, the granuloma often arising on the buccal aspect from the interdental papilla, originating especially where there is a slight malocclusion leading to plaque accumulation.

252

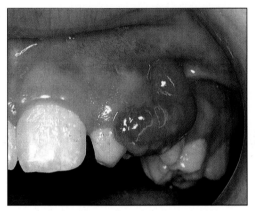

252 A large vascular fibroepithelial polyp arising from the interdental area between a maxillary primary canine and primary first molar. The first molar had extensive mesial caries.

253

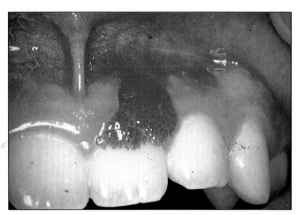

253 Pyogenic granuloma.

254

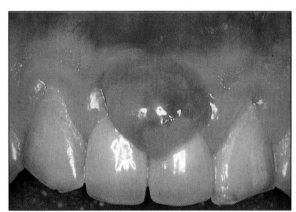

254 Pyogenic granuloma arising from the anterior maxillary gingiva in a patient with very poor oral hygiene.

Giant cell granuloma (giant cell epulis)

Giant cell granuloma (255) is most common in children, and presents as a non-neoplastic swelling of proliferating fibroblasts in a highly vascular stroma containing many multinucleate giant cells.

The giant cell epulis characteristically arises interdentally, adjacent to permanent teeth which have had predecessors, i.e. not the permanent molars. Traditionally, the most notable feature is the deep-red colour, although older lesions tend to be paler. This is a benign lesion.

Giant cell granulomas are *occasionally* a feature of hyperparathyroidism.

255

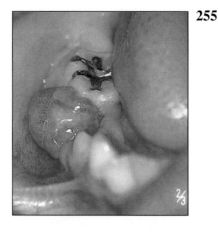

255 Giant cell granuloma.

Lateral periodontal abscess (parodontal abscess)

256

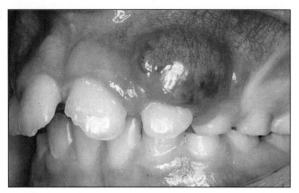

Lateral periodontal abscesses (256) are seen almost exclusively in patients with chronic periodontitis, but may follow impaction of a foreign body, or are related to a lateral root canal on a non-vital tooth. Debris and pus cannot easily escape from the pocket and therefore an acute abscess, with pain and swelling, results.

Lateral periodontal abscesses usually discharge either through the pocket or buccally, but more coronal than a periapical abscess.

256 Lateral periodonal abscess.

Periodontitis

Chronic periodontitis (257) is rare in children. Related to plaque accumulation, it progresses from marginal gingivitis. The features are those of marginal gingivitis but, with destruction of alveolar bone support, there is deep pocket formation and associated tooth mobility and migration.

Accelerated (prepubertal) periodontitis is also rare in children. In this instance, periodontitis develops despite good control of plaque and it is typically related to an immune defect. A range of systemic causes may underlie this accelerated periodontitis, notably poorly controlled diabetes mellitus, white cell dyscrasias including neutrophil defects and neutropenias, and other immune defects including AIDS and Papillon–Lefévre syndrome (268, 349).

Localised juvenile periodontitis is characterised by localised periodontal destruction, classically in the permanent incisor and first molar regions in adolescents or young adults in the absence of poor oral hygiene or gross systemic disease.

Juvenile periodontitis (periodontosis) occurs in females in particular, and may be associated with minor defects of neutrophil function, and with microorganisms such as *Actinobacillus* (haemophilus) *actinomycetemcomitans* and capnocytophaga. Similar periodontal destruction can be seen in Down's syndrome, type VIII Ehlers–Danlos syndrome, and hypophosphatasia.

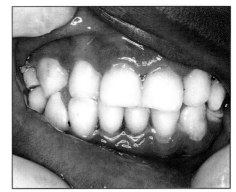

257 Periodontitis affecting the maxillary and mandibular labial segments in a 9-year-old child with poor oral hygiene and a history of previous episodes of ANG.

Trauma

Self-induced ulcers of the gingival margin are not common, but may be seen in disturbed children. The upper canine region buccally seems a typical site for damage by picking with the fingernails.

Trauma (**258–261**) can damage the periodontium, sometimes through excessive occlusal stresses and sometimes through direct damage (class II division 2 malocclusion). In this malocclusion, the upper incisors can strip the periodontium labial to the lower incisors, while the upper incisor periodontium may be traumatised palatally by the lower incisors.

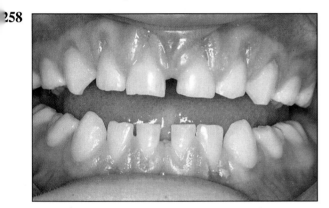

258 Gingivitis artefacta produced by the fingernails in a 6-year-old child. The maxillary anterior gingivae are the most severely affected. There is recession of the gingival margins and the root surfaces are visible.

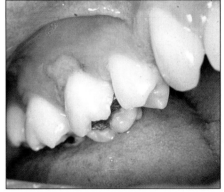

259 Gingival damage produced by a fingernail.

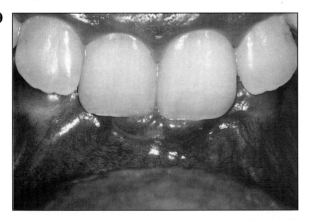

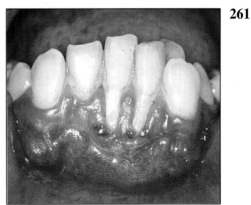

260, 261 Gingival damage as a consequence of a class II division 2 malocclusion (**260**), and with a deep overbite (**261**).

5. Acquired Mucosal Disorders

Acquired immune deficiency syndrome (AIDS, HIV-related disease)

Infection with human immunodeficiency viruses (HIV) may cause an initial glandular fever-like illness but may be asymptomatic. The incubation period may extend over five or more years, during which time certain T lymphocytes (CD_4 cells) are damaged, predisposing to viral, fungal and some other infections. Oral candidosis (262–264), especially thrush and erythematous candidosis, is seen in over 60% of patients, often as an early manifestation, is the most common oral feature of HIV-related disease and may be a predictor of other opportunistic infections and of oesophageal thrush. Other types of oral candidosis may be seen, including angular stomatitis. Xerostomia may predispose to candidosis and also to dental caries.

Kaposi's sarcoma is a rare feature of childhood AIDS: oral lesions are macules or nodules, red to purple in colour and most common in the palate.

Hairy leukoplakia of the tongue is seen in some patients. This lesion is not known to be premalignant but it is a predictor of bad prognosis. The leukoplakia may be corrugated (or 'hairy') and usually affects the lateral margins of the tongue. Hairy leukoplakia may be associated with Epstein–Barr virus and may resolve with antiviral agents such as acyclovir. Occasionally, it is seen in other immunocompromised patients.

Recurrent herpes simplex infection may be labial or intraoral, presenting as chronic ulcers. Cytomegalovirus may also cause ulcers (265).

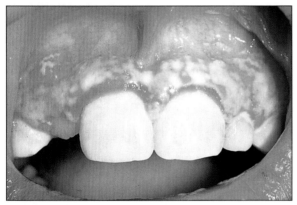

262 Oral candidosis in HIV disease, showing typical lesions of thrush (pseudomembraneous candidiosis).

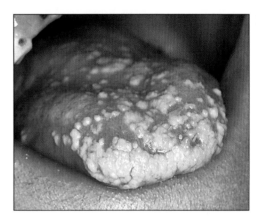

263 Oral candidosis (thrush) in HIV disease.

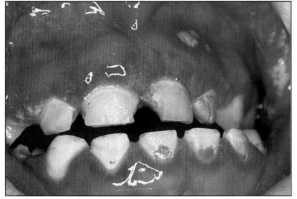

264 Oral erythematous candidosis and neglect, with extensive caries in HIV disease.

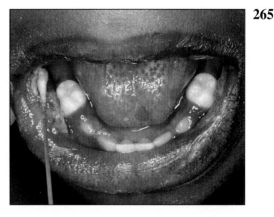

265 Intraoral herpetic ulceration in the buccal mucosa in a patient with AIDS who also has oral candidiosis

Other oral viral infections include human papillomavirus (HPV) infections.

Necrotising gingivitis and destructive periodontitis are occasional features of HIV infection (**266–269**). Aphthous-type ulcers, especially of the major type, may appear in HIV disease. Mouth ulcers are also occasionally caused by other opportunistic pathogens such as mycobacteria and, rarely, by histoplasma or cryptococcus. Other oral or perioral lesions in HIV infection include cervical lymph node enlargement, lymphomas (particularly non-Hodgkin's lymphomas), petechiae, cranial neuropathies and parotitis (**270**).

Intrauterine infection may result in enamel hypoplasia and may cause facial dysmorphogenesis and a foetal AIDS syndrome—though this is controversial.

266

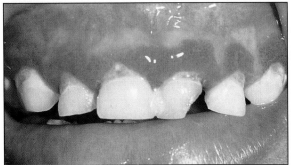

266 HIV disease: gingivitis, and caries.

267

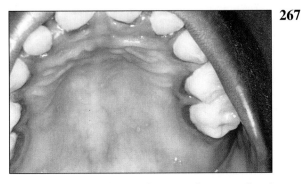

267 HIV-gingivitis showing linear erythematous band at the gingival margin and good oral hygiene.

268

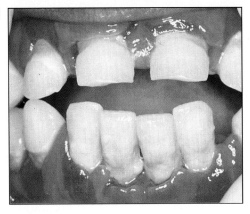

268 HIV periodontitis.

269

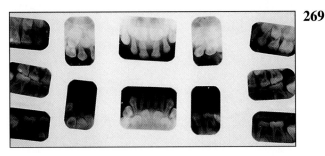

269 HIV periodontitis: radiographs showing alveolar bone loss.

270

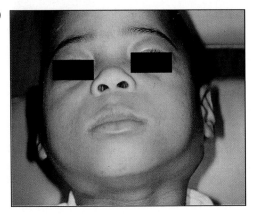

270 HIV salivary gland disease affecting predominantly the parotid glands.

Acute candidosis (thrush, candidiasis, acute pseudomembranous candidosis, moniliasis)

Candida species are common oral commensals. *Candida albicans* is the most common species, which can act as an opportunistic pathogen if the oral ecology is disturbed in xerostomia or by corticosteorids or antibiotics, or if the patient is immunocompromised.

Thrush appears as white flecks or plaques (**262–264, 271**), which are easily removed with gauze to leave an erythematous base. Thrush can affect any oral site, typically the palate or upper buccal vestibule posteriorly. Acute candidosis can also present as red lesions (erythematous candidosis).

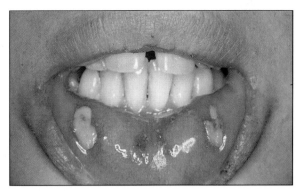

271

271 Thrush in a leukaemic patient.

Amalgam and other tattoos

Amalgam tattoos are common causes of blue-black pigmentation (**272, Table 6**), and are usually seen buccally in the mandibular gingiva, or at least close to the teeth, mainly in older children or adolescents. Radio-opacities may or may not be seen on radiography. Similar lesions can result if for some reason pencil lead or other similar foreign bodies become embedded in the oral tissues.

Radiography may help to confirm the diagnosis. Biopsy may be indicated to exclude a naevus or melanoma, but otherwise these lesions are innocuous.

Occasionally, adolescents may have tattoos made in their mouth deliberately (**273**).

Table 6 Main causes of oral pigmentation in childhood.

DISCRETE AREAS

Amalgam tattoo
Ephelis (freckle)
Naevus
Laugier–Hunziker syndrome
Melanotic macules
Complex of myxomas, spotty pigmentation and
 endocrine overactivity
Malignant melanoma
Kaposi's sarcoma
Peutz–Jeghers syndrome

GENERALISED

Racial
Drugs, e.g. antimalarials, minocycline
Addison's disease
Albright's syndrome
Other rare causes, e.g. haemochromatosis,
 generalised neurofibromatosis, incontinentia pigmenti

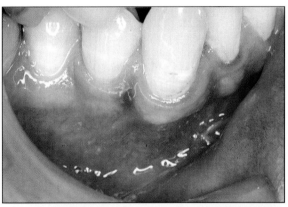

272

273

272 Amalgam tattoo.

273 Deliberate intra-oral tattoo.

Angular stomatitis (angular cheilitis, cheilosis, perléche)

274

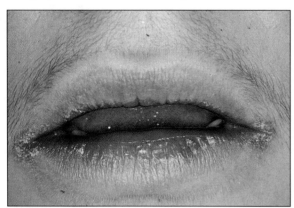

Angular stomatitis is bilateral and produces erythema, fissuring or ulceration which can be painful and disfiguring (**274**). Rarely, angular stomatitis is a manifestation of iron deficiency or of vitamin deficiency such as in Crohn's disease (*see* p. 89)—when there may also be glossitis and mouth ulcers—or of an immune defect (**351**). Although *Candida albicans* is the prevalent organism, *Staphylococcus aureus* and other microorganisms may sometimes be isolated.

274 Angular stomatitis in a diabetic patient.

Aphthae (recurrent aphthous stomatitis, RAS)

Mouth ulcers may have a range of causes (**Tables 7** and **8**). Aphthae are typically recurrent, ovoid or round ulcers with a yellowish floor and pronounced red inflammatory halo. Episodes begin usually in childhood and the natural history is of spontaneous remission after some years.

Minor aphthae (**275**) (Mikulcz aphthae) are small, 2–4 mm in diameter, last 7–10 days, tend not to be seen on the gingiva, palate or dorsum of the tongue, and heal with no obvious scarring. Most patients develop no more than six ulcers in any single episode.

Major aphthae (**276**) are recurrent, often ovoid ulcers with an inflammatory halo, but are less common, much larger, and more persistent than minor aphthae, and can affect the dorsum of the tongue and soft palate as well as other sites. Sometimes termed Sutton's ulcers or periadenitis mucosa necrotica recurrens (PMNR), major aphthae can be well over 1 cm in diameter and can take several months to heal. At any one episode there are usually fewer than six ulcers present. Major aphthae may leave obvious scars on healing.

Herpetiform aphthae are so termed because the patients have a myriad of small ulcers that clinically resemble those of herpetic stomatitis. Herpetiform aphthae are, however, a distinct entity, lacking the associated fever, gingivitis and regional lymphadenopathy of primary herpetic stomatitis. Pinpoint herpetiform aphthae enlarge and fuse to produce irregular ulcers. The aetiology of aphthae is unknown. Most patients with RAS are otherwise apparently well, but a significant proportion of those referred to a hospital clinic prove to be deficient in a haematinic such as iron, folate or vitamin B_{12}. About 2–3% have coeliac disease, and there are also occasional associations with stress, food allergy, and immunodeficiencies including HIV disease.

Aphthae may occasionally be associated with menstruation, and may be a manifestation of Behçet's syndrome (*see* p. 85). Aphthous-like ulcers may also occasionally be a manifestation of cyclic neutropenia, or a similar recently described syndrome with periodic fever and pharyngitis, but with no neutropenia.

Table 7 Main causes of mouth ulcers in children.

Local causes (e.g. trauma)
Recurrent aphthae (and Behçet's syndrome)
Malignant neoplasms (rarely)
Ulcers associated with systemic disease (e.g. coeliac disease)
Drugs (e.g. cytotoxics)
Irradiation of the oral mucosa

Table 8 Main causes of mouth ulcers associated with systemic disease in children.

Microbial disease

>   Herpetic stomatitis
>   Chickenpox
>   Hand, foot and mouth disease
>   Herpangina
>   Infectious mononucleosis
>   Acute necrotising gingivitis
>   HIV infection
>   Rarely: fungal infections, tuberculosis or syphilis

Malignant neoplasms (rarely)

Cutaneous disease (uncommon)

>   Erosive lichen planus
>   Pemphigus
>   Pemphigoid
>   Erythema multiforme
>   Dermatitis herpetiformis and linear IgA disease
>   Epidermolysis bullosa
>   Other dermatoses

Blood disorders

>   Anaemia
>   Leukaemia
>   Neutropenia
>   Other white cell dyscrasias

Gastrointestinal disease

>   Coeliac disease
>   Crohn's disease
>   Ulcerative colitis

Rheumatic diseases (rarely)

>   Lupus erythematosus
>   Behçet's syndrome
>   Sweet's syndrome

Drugs

>   Cytotoxic and other agents
>   Acrodynia

Radiotherapy

Disorders of uncertain pathogenesis

>   Eosinophilic ulcer
>   Necrotising sialometaplasia

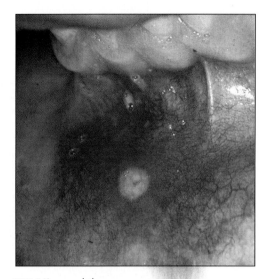

275

275 Minor aphthae.

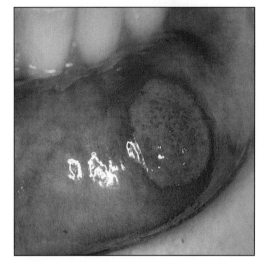

276

276 Major aphthae.

Aplastic anaemia

Clinical features of aplastic anaemia depend on the predominant bone marrow cell type affected and therefore there may be features of thrombocytopenia, leucopenia, anaemia (**277, 278**) or a combination (pancytopenia). Spontaneous purpuric or ecchymotic haemorrhages of the skin and mucous membrane are the common presenting features (**279**). Leucopenia (particularly neutropenia) leads to decreased resistance to infection, and manifests as severe oral ulceration, often associated with opportunistic organisms. Typically there is, as in agranulocytosis, only a minimal red inflammatory halo around the ulcers.

Bone marrow transplantation (BMT) is often the treatment for aplastic anaemia and may present oral complications including mucositis, candidosis, parotitis, graft-versus-host disease with lichenoid or sclerodermatous reactions, or infections with herpesviruses or fungi, such as aspergillus (*see* p. 88). Xerostomia predisposes to caries.

277

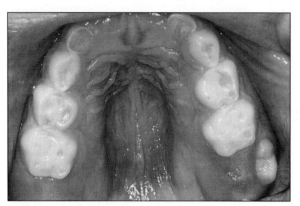

277 Palatal bruising in a patient with aplastic anaemia and thrombocytopenia.

278

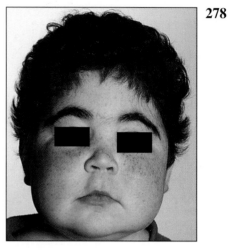

278 Systemic corticosteroid therapy for the patient in **277** has resulted in hirsutism and a rounding of the facial features—so-called `moon face'.

279

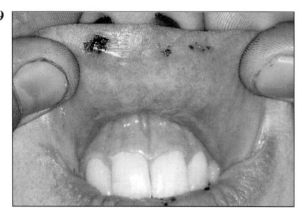

279 Oral purpura. Similar lesions are not infrequently seen because of trauma in healthy persons. N.B. Clinicians must now always wear gloves during patient care.

Behçet's syndrome (Behçet's disease)

Aphthae of any of the types described above (*see* p. 82) usually occur in isolation in apparently healthy persons (**280**). A minority are a manifestation of Behçet's syndrome, where aphthae are associated with genital ulcers and uveitis. Behçet's syndrome is more common in adults, and in Japan, China, Korea and the Middle East, and may have an immunogenetic basis.

Behçet's syndrome is a multisystem disease affecting the mouth in most cases. Other sites commonly affected are genitals, eyes, skin and joints (**281**); but Behçet's syndrome is not the only cause of this constellation of lesions. Others include ulcerative colitis, Crohn's disease, mixed connective tissue disease, lupus erythematosus and Reiter's syndrome, which should all be excluded.

Uveitis (posterior uveitis; retinal vasculitis) is one of the more important ocular lesions of Behçet's syndrome but anterior uveitis and other changes can occur. Ocular symptoms are more common in males. Neurological involvement may cause headache, psychiatric, motor or sensory manifestations.

Of the various rashes seen in Behçet's syndrome, an acneiform pustular rash is common, and patients may develop pustules at the site of venepuncture (pathergy). However, this feature is uncommon in British patients. Erythema nodosum can be a feature of Behçet's syndrome, particularly in females. Large joint arthropathy is not uncommon in Behçet's syndrome (**282**), but an overlap syndrome with relapsing polychondritis has also been described (mouth and genital ulcers with inflamed cartilage (MAGIC) syndrome).

280

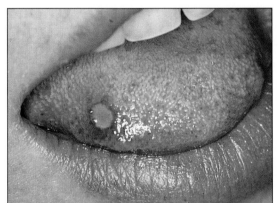

280 Aphthae in Behçet's syndrome.

281

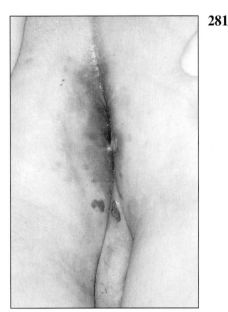

281 Perianal ulceration in Behçet's syndrome.

282

282 Erythema nodosum in Behçet's syndrome.

Burns

Burns (**283–289**) are most common after the ingestion of hot foods and are seen particularly on the palate or tongue, for example, 'pizza-palate'. Some patients attempt to relieve oral pain by holding an analgesic tablet at the site of pain. Aspirin has commonly produced burns. X-irradiation may produce burns.

Cold injury is uncommon, but follows cryosurgery. Actinic burns are uncommon in children. Electrical burns are also uncommon, seen usually in pre-school children who bite electric flex. Very rarely, burns are caused by caustic liquid or natural products such as the houseplant dieffenbachia, or the enzyme bromelin in pineapple.

283

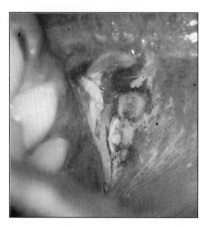

283 Cotton wool burn of the maxillary labial sulcus.

284

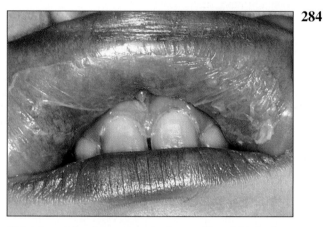

284 A burn/allergic response in the maxillary labial sulcus that appeared shortly after using lignocaine topical gel prior to infiltration anaesthetic.

285

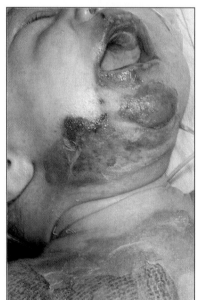

286

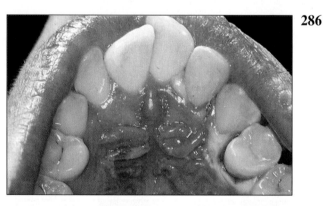

286 Burn of the palatal mucosa caused by dentine primer that had leaked under a rubber dam.

285 Burns of the lips, premaxilla, chin, neck and thorax of a baby who had reached up on to a table and pulled a pot of freshly made hot tea over himself.

287

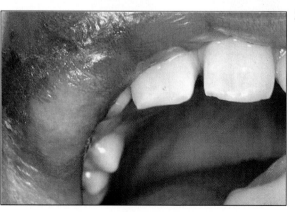

287 A handpiece burn of the upper lip after restoration of a maxillary molar.

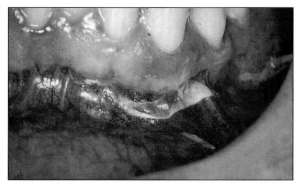

288 Chemical burn from mouthwash use.

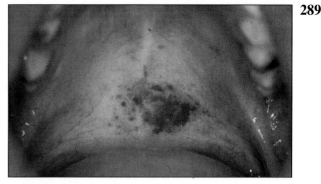

289 Petechiae after eating an ice lollipop.

Cheek-chewing (morsicatio buccarum)

Cheek- or lip-biting (**290**) is often a neurotic trait. The mucosa is shredded with a shaggy white appearance similar to that of white sponge naevus (**143**) but restricted to areas close to the occlusal line.

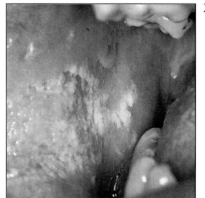

290 Cheek-biting (morsicatio buccarum).

Chemotherapy-induced mucosal and other lesions

There are immediate haemorrhagic, infective and ulcerative oral complications of chemotherapy, which resolve once treatment is finished (**291–299**). Long-term effects, however, are recorded in the teeth that were mineralising when chemotherapy was given and include crown abnormalities (hypoplasia, microdontia or taurodontism) and root anomalies (shortened, constricted, tapered or thinned). Teeth may also fail to develop.

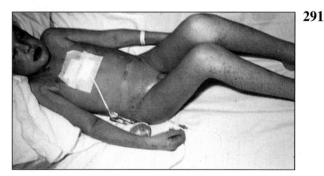

291 Fulminant septicaemia of oral origin in a child undergoing chemotherapy.

292

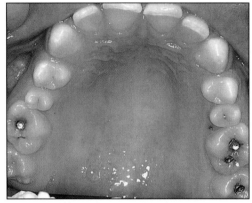

292 Enamel hypoplasia in a child who received cancer chemotherapy for acute lymphoblastic leukaemia from 2–4$\frac{1}{2}$ years of age.

293

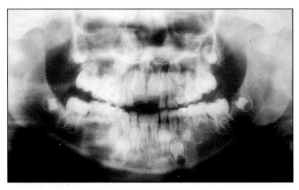

293 Microdontia of developing second permanent molars. Chemotherapy was given from 1–3 years of age for an embryonal yolk sac tumour.

294

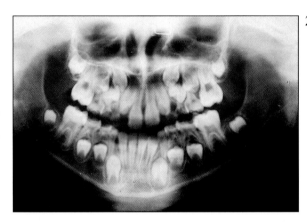

294 Erupted microdont maxillary second premolars. This patient received chemotherapy for acute lymphoblastic leukaemia for 2$\frac{1}{2}$ years from the age of 1$\frac{1}{2}$.

295

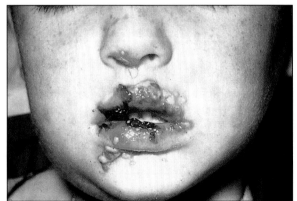

295 Microdont second permanent molars and taurodont first permanent molars in a child who received chemotherapy for acute lymphoblastic leukaemia for 2$\frac{1}{2}$ years from the age of 2.

296

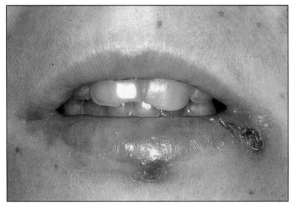

297

296, 297 Herpes simplex virus infection in children undergoing cancer chemotherapy.

298

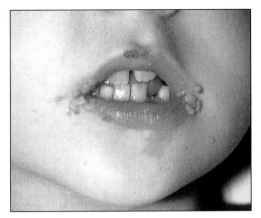

298 Papillomavirus infection in a child undergoing cancer chemotherapy.

299

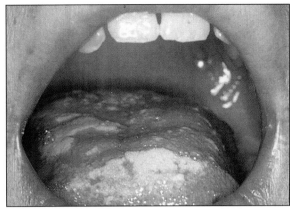

299 Candidosis (thrush) in a child undergoing cancer chemotherapy.

Crohn's disease and orofacial granulomatosis

Crohn's disease is a chronic inflammatory bowel disease of unknown aetiology, affecting mainly the ileum. However, any part of the gastrointestinal tract can be involved, including the mouth (**300–308**). The majority of patients with 'oral Crohn's disease' do not, however, have identifiable gastrointestinal lesions. Non-caseating granulomas are seen in oral Crohn's disease but similar cases are related to allergies such as those to food constituents like cinnamaldehyde (the term 'orofacial granulomatosis' is then often used) or sarcoidosis. Swelling of the lips and angular stomatitis are common. Persistent irregular oral ulcers or classic aphthae are common features. Gingival swelling may be a feature and oral mucosal tags are seen in some patients. Folding of the oral mucosa may lead to a 'cobblestone' appearance.

Melkersson–Rosenthal syndrome, a related condition, is discussed on p. 35.

300

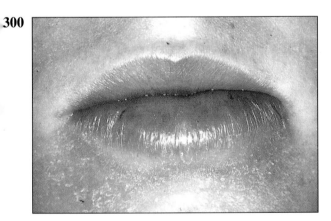

300 Labial swelling in orofacial granulomatosis.

301

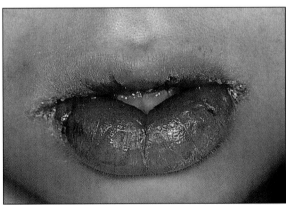

301 Labial swelling, fissuring and angular stomatitis in orofacial granulomatosis.

302

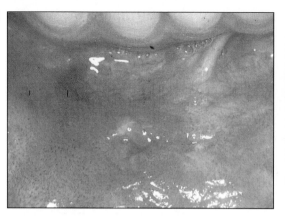

302 Oral ulceration in orofacial granulomatosis.

303

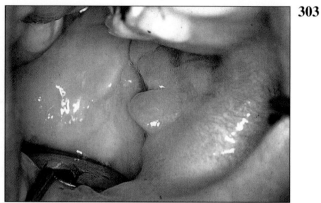

303 Cobblestoning of the buccal mucosa in orofacial granulomatosis.

304

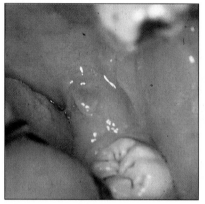

304 Mucosal tags in orofacial granulomatosis.

305

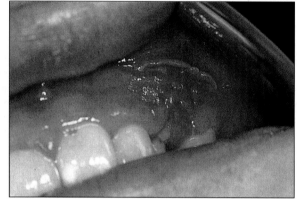

305 Gingival proliferative lesions in orofacial granulomatosis.

306

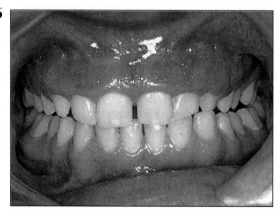

306 Gingival lesions in orofacial granulomatosis.

307

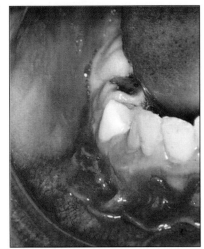

308

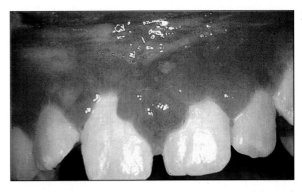

307, 308 Gingival swelling and cobblestoning of the oral mucosa of two children with orofacial granulomatosis.

Deep mycoses

The deep mycoses are rare in children. Despite the fact that Rhizopus, Mucor and Absidia are fungi ubiquitous in decaying vegetation and some sugary foods, zygomycosis (phycomycosis; mucormycosis) is rare and seen almost exclusively in immunocompromised patients (**309**). Nasal and paranasal sinus zygomycosis is seen in poorly controlled diabetics, and it may invade the orbit, frontal lobe, palate and elsewhere.

Aspergillosis, infection with aspergillosis species, usually with *Aspergillus fumigatus*, but also *A. flavus* and *A. niger*, can present in several ways. The most serious is systemic aspergillosis, or respiratory tract aspergillus infection in immunocompromised patients. In aspergillus sinusitis, there are normally non-invasive fungus balls, but infection of the antrum may rarely invade the palate, orbit or brain. It has been reported that antral aspergillosis can be precipitated by overfilling maxillary root canals with endodontic material containing zinc oxide and paraformaldehyde.

Other deep mycoses are seen mainly in the endemic areas, predominantly in the tropics, and in adults.

309

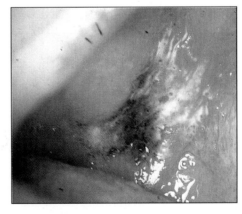

309 Deep mycosis in a leukaemic patient.

Dog bites

310

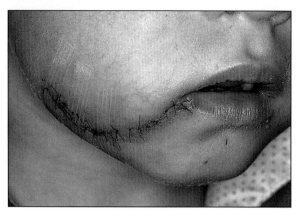

Dogs occasionally, and other animals—or even humans rarely—can inflict bites around the mouth (**310**). Animal bites may become infected by unusual micro-organisms.

310 Severe orofacial wound from a dog bite, after repair.

Erythema multiforme

Although the aetiology of erythema multiforme is unclear in most patients, in some this mucocutaneous disorder is precipitated by infections (such as herpes simplex or mycoplasma), by drugs (sulphonamides, barbiturates, hydantoins and others), or by a range of other triggers.

Most patients are males, typically adolescents or young adults, and there are periods of remission from the disease. The virtually pathognomonic feature of erythema multiforme is swollen, blood-stained or crusted lips (**311**).

Oral lesions progress through macules to blisters and ulcers, typically most pronounced in the anterior parts of the mouth. Extensive oral ulceration may be seen (**312**).

Most patients have oral lesions only, but in some, other squamous epithelia are involved. Rashes of various types (hence 'erythema multiforme') are seen. The characteristic rash consists of 'target' or 'iris' lesions in which the central lesion has a surrounding ring of erythema (**313**).

Conjunctivitis, stomatitis and rash occur together in Stevens–Johnson syndrome (erythema multiforme exudativum). The ocular changes resemble those of mucous membrane pemphigoid: dry eyes and symblepharon may result. Balanitis, urethritis and vulval ulcers are typical genital lesions.

311

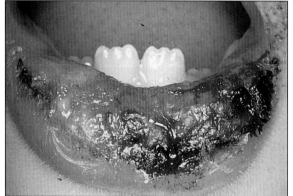

311 Labial swelling and blood-stained crusting of a young boy with oral erythema multiforme.

312

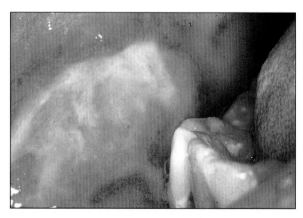

312 Oral erosions in erythema multiforme.

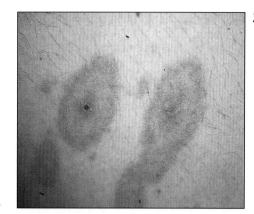

313 Typical target or iris rash of erythema multiforme.

Furred tongue

The tongue is rarely furred in a healthy child. Any febrile illness may cause a furred tongue (**314**).

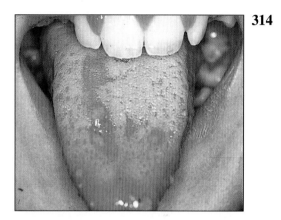

314 Furred tongue in an ill child—in this case primary herpetic stomatitis (ulceration is also evident).

Gluten-sensitive enteropathy (coeliac disease)

Up to 3% of patients seen as out-patients with aphthae prove to have coeliac disease (**315, 316**). Other oral manifestations may include glossitis, angular stomatitis and dental hypoplasia.

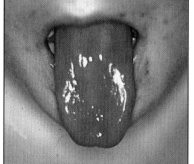

315 Glossitis in coeliac disease.

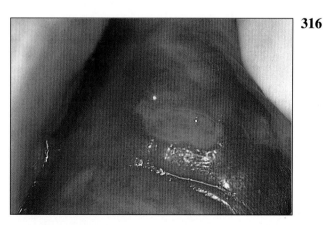

316 Aphthous ulceration in coeliac disease.

Hand, foot and mouth disease (vesicular stomatitis with exanthem)

317

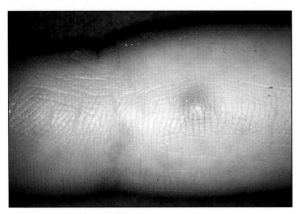

317 Vesicles in hand, foot and mouth disease.

This Coxsackie virus infection produces small painful vesicles surrounded by inflammatory haloes, especially on the dorsum and lateral aspect of the fingers and toes (**317**). Coxsackie virus A16 is usually implicated, but A5, A7, A9 and A10, or viruses of the B9 group, or other enteroviruses, may be responsible.

The incubation period is up to a week. A rash is not always present or may affect more proximal parts of the limbs or buttocks. The vesicles usually heal spontaneously in about one week.

Oral lesions are non-specific, usually affecting the tongue or buccal mucosa. Ulcers are shallow, painful and very small, surrounded by inflammatory haloes.

Reports of other systemic manifestations such as encephalitis are very rare, except in enterovirus 71 infection.

Herpangina

318

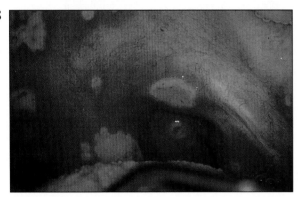

318 Palatal ulceration of herpangina.

Herpangina is usually caused by Coxsackie viruses A1–A6, A8, A10, A12 or A22, but similar syndromes can be caused by other viruses, especially Coxsackie B and echoviruses. Herpangina presents with fever, malaise, headache, and a sore throat caused by an ulcerating vesicular eruption in the oropharynx. Vesicles rupture to leave painful, shallow, round ulcers, mainly on the fauces and soft palate (**318**). These heal spontaneously in 7–10 days.

Faucial ulcers, sometimes with a rash and aseptic meningitis, are characteristic of echovirus 9 infection. Lesions resembling Koplik's spots (**345**) may be seen in echovirus 9 infections, along with a rash and aseptic meningitis.

Herpes simplex virus (HSV) infections

319

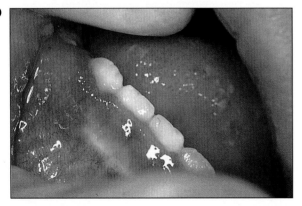

319 Gingival swelling and erythema in primary herpetic stomatitis.

Herpetic stomatitis is typically a childhood infection seen between the ages of 2–4 years, after an incubation period of approximately 6–7 days. Gingival oedema, erythema and ulceration are prominent features of primary infection, which is usually caused by HSV-1.

Widespread oral vesicles break down to leave pin-point ulcers that enlarge and fuse to produce irregular painful oral ulcers. Herpetic stomatitis (**319–321**) probably explains many instances of 'teething'. Patients can be severely ill, with malaise, fever and cervical lymph node enlargement. The tongue is often coated and there is halitosis. Rarely, acute necrotising gingivitis follows. The saliva is heavily infected with HSV, which may cause lip and skin lesions and is a source for cross-infection.

Rare complications of HSV infection include encephalitis and mononeuropathies. HSV remains latent in the trigeminal ganglion and reactivation—for example, by fever, sunlight, trauma or immunosuppression—can produce herpes labialis (**296, 297, 322, 323**). Some 6–14% of the population have a recurrent HSV infection. It presents as macules that rapidly become papular and vesicular, typically at the mucocutaneous junction of the lip. Lesions then become pustular, scab and heal without scarring.

Herpes simplex infection due to reactivation of latent HSV is rare intraorally, but may follow the trauma of a local anaesthetic injection or be seen in immuno-compromised patients. Recurrent intraoral herpes in normal patients thus tends to affect the hard palate or gingiva and heals within 1–2 weeks. Immunocompromised patients may develop chronic, often dendritic, ulcers, frequently on the tongue. Clinical diagnosis tends to underestimate the frequency of these lesions.

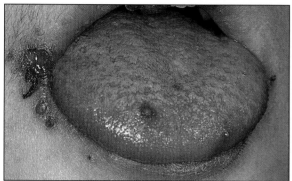

320 Ulcers on tongue, and skin lesions, in primary herpetic stomatitis.

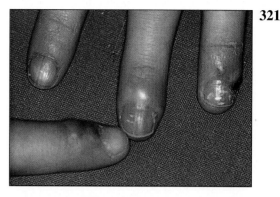

321 Lesions on skin resulting from contamination by infected saliva in primary herpetic stomatitis.

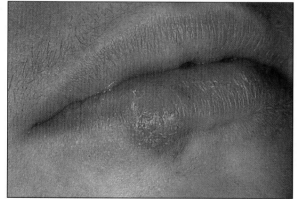

322 Herpes labialis at a typical site.

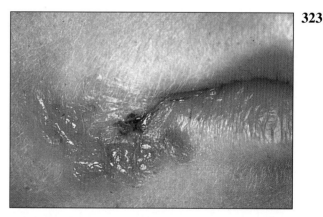

323 Herpes labialis at the right angle of the mouth. The vesicular lesions have burst to leave a scab that will heal without scarring.

Human papillomavirus infections

Human papillomavirus (HPV) infections cause verruca vulgaris (common wart), condyloma acuminatum (genital wart), papillomas and, rarely, focal epithelial hyperplasia (Heck's disease). HPV lesions are increasingly common, particularly as a complication of HIV disease.

Warts are seen especially on the lips (**298, 324**) or tongue; papillomas are most common on the palate or gingiva. The cauliflower-like appearance of a papilloma is usually obvious (**325, 326**) but may be indis-

tinguishable from a wart. The condyloma acuminatum (genital wart) usually results from orogenital contact and appears as a cauliflower-like lump, mainly in the anterior mouth.

Focal epithelial hyperplasia (Heck's disease) is seen most frequently in Eskimos and North American Indians and presents as multiple painless, sessile, soft papules, generally whitish in colour, usually in the buccal or lower labial mucosa.

324

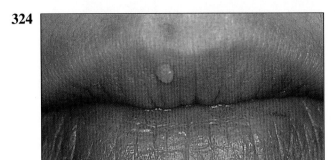

324 Wart on the lip.

325

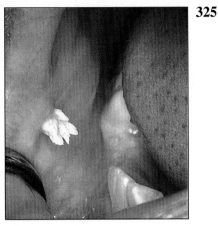

325 Papilloma of the oral mucosa just inside the right commissure.

326

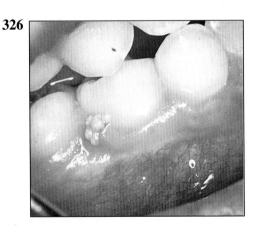

326 Gingival papilloma.

Iatrogenic injury

Haematomas may be produced by trauma, such as by dental local anaesthetic injections, especially regional blocks. They are usually inconsequential unless intramuscular, when they can cause trismus, or become infected. Occasionally after tooth extraction blood may track through the fascial planes of the neck to cause extensive bruising, even down to the chest wall. Iatrogenic oral ulceration can be produced by trauma (**327**), burns, and chemicals.

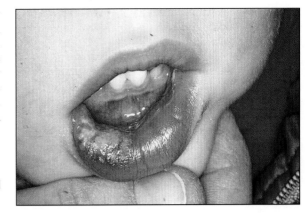

327

327 Ulcer from biting the lower lip. N.B. Gloves should now always be worn during patient care.

Infectious mononucleosis (Paul–Bunnell positive glandular fever)

Infectious mononucleosis (IM) is caused by the Epstein–Barr virus (EBV), and is more common in the West in teenagers and young adults than in young children. The incubation period of 30–50 days is followed by fever, sore throat and lymph node enlargement; mouth ulcers may be seen together with faucial oedema and tonsillar exudate (**328**). There is severe dysphagia, and faucial oedema can, rarely, obstruct the airway.

Palatal petechiae (**329**), especially at the junction of the hard and soft palate, are almost pathognomonic of IM but can be seen in other viral infections such as HIV and rubella, and in non-infective causes of thrombocytopathy.

A feature that may suggest IM is the occurrence of a rash if the patient is given ampicillin or amoxycillin (this may also be seen in lymphoid leukaemias). The rash is often morbilliform and does not represent penicillin allergy. A few patients develop a maculopapular rash even if not taking synthetic penicillins.

EBV may also cause persistent malaise, and has associations with Duncan's disease (X-linked lymphoproliferative syndrome), Burkitt's lymphoma and other neoplasms, and hairy leukoplakia.

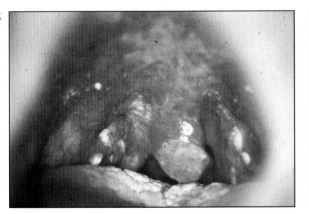

328

328 Faucial oedema, exudate and ulceration in infectious mononucleosis.

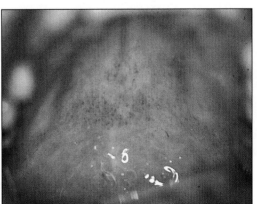

329

329 Palatal petechiae in infectious mononucleosis.

Langerhan's cell histiocytoses

Langerhan's cell histiocytoses are a group of disorders, formerly termed histiocytosis X, arising from Langerhan's cells (**330–333**).

Letterer–Siwe disease is an acute disseminated and usually lethal form of histiocytosis seen in children under the age of 3 years. There are bone lesions, mucocutaneous lesions, fever, lymphadenopathy and hepatosplenomegaly.

Hand–Schüller–Christian disease appears at 3–6 years of age with osteolytic jaw lesions and loosening of teeth ('floating teeth'), diabetes insipidus and exophthalmos.

Eosinophilic granuloma is a localised benign form of histiocytosis typically seen in older patients, where there are painless osteolytic bone lesions and, sometimes, mouth ulcers. The affected teeth may loosen.

330

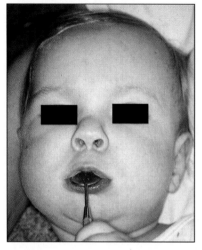

330 Facial swelling in Langerhan's histiocytosis.

331

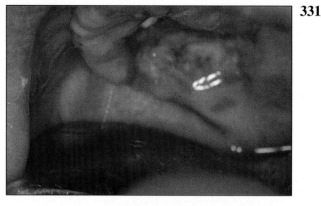

331 Palatal swelling in Langerhan's histiocytosis.

332

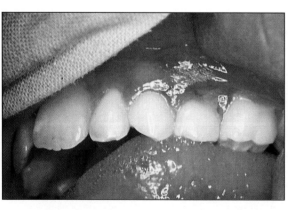

332 Gingival ulceration in Langerhan's histiocytosis.

333

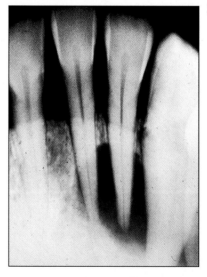

333 Radiolucent lesion ('floating teeth') in Langerhan's histiocytosis.

Leukaemias

Spontaneous gingival haemorrhage and oral purpura are common in leukaemia, but there are no oral features that distinguish reliably between the different leukaemias (**334–337**) and gingival bleeding has other causes (**Table 9**).

Oral purpura is seen particularly where there is trauma, and chemotherapy may aggravate the bleeding tendency. Gingival haemorrhage can be so profuse as to dissuade the patient from oral hygiene, but this simply aggravates the problem as the gingivae then become inflamed, more hyperaemic and bleed more profusely. Mouth ulcers are common in leukaemia. Some are associated with chemotherapy, some with viral, bacterial or fungal infection, and some are non-specific.

Leukaemic deposits in the gingiva occasionally cause gingival swelling, a feature especially of myelomonocytic leukaemia.

Microbial infections—mainly fungal and viral—are common in the mouth and can be a significant problem to the leukaemic patient. Candidosis is extremely common but aspergillosis and zygomycosis are fortunately rare. Of the viral infections, recurrent intraoral herpes simplex is also common.

Recurrent herpes labialis is common in leukaemic patients. The lesions can be extensive and, because of the thrombocytopenia, there is often bleeding into the lesions.

Simple odontogenic infections can spread widely and be difficult to control. Non-odontogenic oral infections are common in leukaemic patients and can involve a range of bacteria including *Staphylococcus aureus*, *Pseudomonas aeruginosa*, *Klebsiella pneumoniae*, *Staphylococcus epidermidis*, *Escherichia coli*, and enterococci.

334

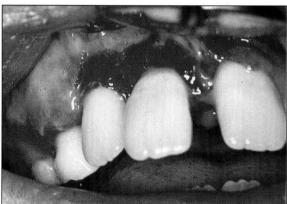

334 Gingival purpura in acute lymphoblastic leukaemia.

335 Purpura in leukaemia.

335

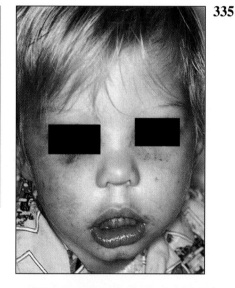

336

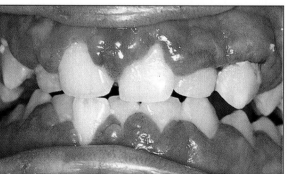

337

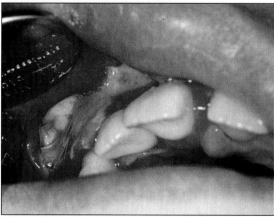

336 Gingival swelling in myelomonocytic leukaemia.

337 Oral ulceration in acute lymphoblastic leukaemia.

Table 9 Causes of gingival bleeding in childhood.

LOCAL

Acute necrotising gingivitis
Chronic gingivitis
Chronic periodontitis

SYSTEMIC

Any thrombocytopathy
Leukaemia
HIV infection
Scurvy
Clotting defects
Drugs, e.g. anticoagulants

Lichenoid lesions and lichen planus

Lichen planus (**338–341**) is rare in children. Usually idiopathic, lesions resembling lichen planus may be drug-induced. Non-steroidal anti-inflammatory agents, and antimalarial drugs are among the causes of lichenoid lesions, as are some restorative materials and graft-versus-host disease.

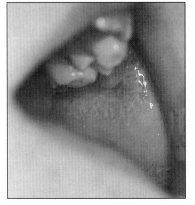

338 Lichen planus (erosive) on the tongue.

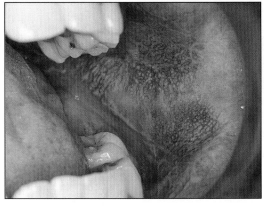

339 Lichen planus with pigmentary incontinence in the buccal mucosa of an Asian patient.

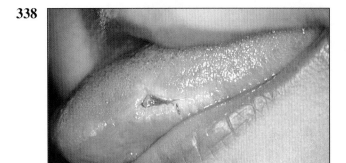

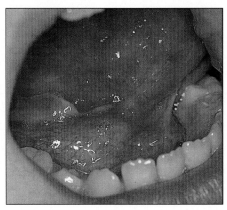

340, 341 Lichen planus in a 10-year-old child, presenting with white lesions and erosions. Lichen planus may present with white lesions, typically in the buccal mucosa bilaterally, and must be distinguished from other oral white lesions (**Table 10**).

Table 10 Main causes of oral white lesions in childhood.

LOCAL

Cheek biting
Frictional keratosis
Burns
Idiopathic keratosis rarely
Carcinoma rarely
Smokeless tobacco use

SYSTEMIC

Candidosis
Lichen planus
Lupus erythematosus
Papillomas (some)
Hairy leukoplakia
Chronic renal failure
Inherited lesions (e.g. white sponge naevus)

Lymphomas

African Burkitt's lymphoma (**342**) is associated with Epstein–Barr virus and typically affects children before the age of 12–13 years. The jaws, particularly the mandible, are common sites of presentation. Massive swelling, which ulcerates in the mouth, may be seen. Radiographically, the teeth may appear to be 'floating in air'.

The association of non-African Burkitt's lymphoma (**343**) with Epstein–Barr virus is tenuous and the disease is less common than the African form. It may cause oral pain, paraesthesia or increasing tooth mobility, but the jaws are less frequently involved in this type of Burkitt's lymphoma. However, discrete radiolucencies in the lower third molar region, destruction of lamina dura and widening of the periodontal space may be seen on radiography.

Other lymphomas are rare in children but, with the increase in HIV disease, are likely to become more common.

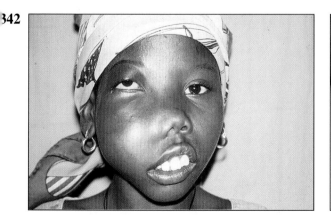

342 African Burkitt's lymphoma showing maxillary involvement.

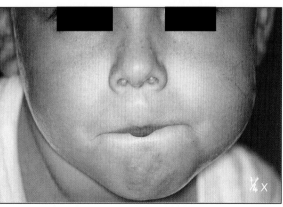

343 Non-African Burkitt's lymphoma involving the mandible.

Measles (rubeola)

Measles is an acute contagious infection with a paramyxovirus. The incubation period of 7–10 days is followed by fever, rhinitis, cough and conjunctivitis (coryza), and then a red maculopapular rash (**344**), which appears initially on the forehead and behind the ears, before spreading over the whole body. Koplik's spots (**345**)—small, whitish, necrotic lesions, said to resemble grains of salt—are found in the buccal mucosa, and occasionally also in the conjunctiva or genitalia, preceding the measles rash by 1–2 days.

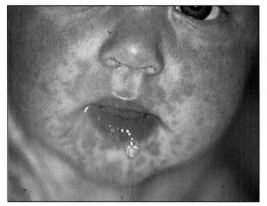

344 Maculopapular rash of measles.

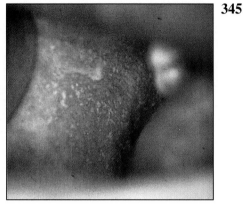

345 Koplik's spots of measles prodrome.

Melanotic naevi

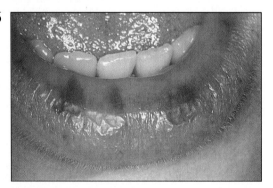

346 Melanotic naevi.

Most intraoral melanotic naevi (**346**) are seen on the hard palate or in the buccal mucosa. The majority are circumscribed, small, greyish or brownish macules and are benign.

The most common are intramucosal naevi. Less common are oral melanotic macules and compound and junctional naevi.

Molluscum contagiosum

Molluscum contagiosum (**347, 348**) is a pox virus infection producing characteristic umbilicated non-tender papules, typically on the skin of male children. Oral lesions, though still very rare, are now being reported in HIV disease. Facial lesions are more common.

347

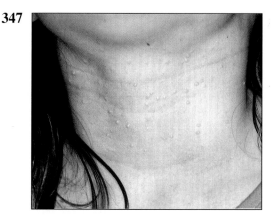

347 Molluscum contagiosum on neck.

348

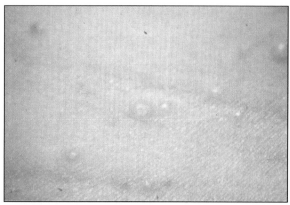

348 Molluscum contagiosum showing umbilicated papules.

Neutrophil disorders

Neutropenias predispose to acute necrotising gingivitis, rapidly destructive periodontal disease and to oral ulceration. Cyclic neutropenia (**349–352**) produces a drop in polymorphonuclear neutrophil count, and sometimes other leukocytes, about every 21 days. Destructive periodontal disease, recurrent necrotising gingivitis and recurrent mouth ulcers are frequent manifestations.

Gangrene may be seen in patients with neutropenia or rare neutrophil defects such as acatalasia (seen mainly in Japan, Korea, Israel and Switzerland).

349

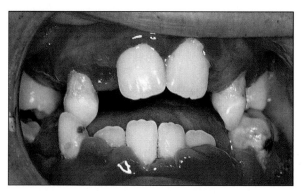

349 Periodontal disease in cyclic neutropenia.

350

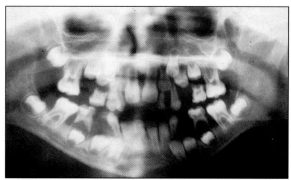

350 Radiograph showing periodontal disease in cyclic neutropenia.

351

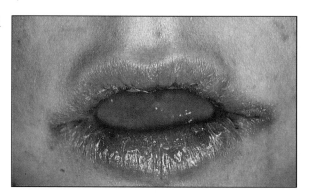

351 Angular stomatitis in cyclic neutropenia.

352

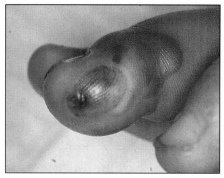

352 Skin infections in cyclic neutropenia.

Pemphigus vulgaris

353

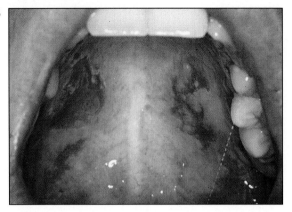

353 Pemphigus affecting the palate of a teenager.

Pemphigus is rare in children but may present with oral erosions, lesions in other mucosae, or skin blisters. It is an autoimmune disease with antibodies directed against the glycoprotein coat of epidermal and mucosal cells, which separate, forming thin-rooted blisters (**353**). The blisters quickly rupture to leave painful erosions. Mouth lesions are an early and prominent feature but may be similar to other forms of oral ulcer and diagnosis is achieved by biopsy, direct immunofluorescence on the biopsy specimen and indirect immunofluorescence technique on the blood. Untreated pemphigus progresses remorselessly and may be fatal. Even with treatment morbidity is severe.

Pyostomatitis vegetans

354

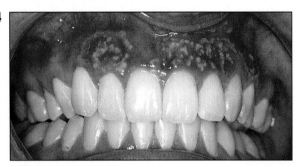

354 Pyostomatitis vegetans in an adolescent with ulcerative colitis.

Reported oral lesions in ulcerative colitis include aphthae, chronic oral ulcers and pyostomatitis vegetans. The course of these lesions tends to follow that of the bowel disease.

Oral lesions termed pyostomatitis vegetans are deep fissures, pustules and papillary projections. Less than 30 cases have been recorded and most patients have had ulcerative colitis (**354**) or Crohn's disease.

Radiotherapy-induced lesions

Mucositis, xerostomia, trismus and loss of taste are almost inevitable after irradiation involving the oral region, though the severity is often related to the radiotherapy regimen used (**355–357**).

Infections (caries, candidosis, acute sialadentitis) and dental hypersensitivity are mainly secondary to reduced salivary function.

Osteoradionecrosis, osteomyelitis and trismus are secondary to endarteritis of the small arteries in bone and muscle.

Radiotherapy involving the jaws may well affect tooth and root development, producing results similar to those seen in patients on cancer chemotherapy.

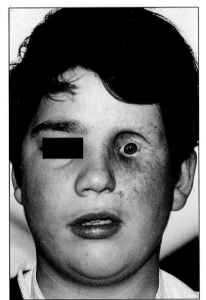

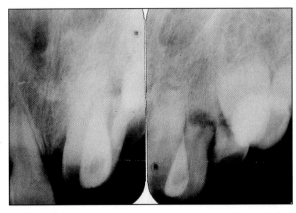

355 Rhabdomyosarcoma of the orbital muscles of the left eye was treated by enucleation and radiotherapy. This has resulted in telangiectasia of the skin of the left side of the eye and cheek and left infraorbital and maxillary hypoplasia.

356 Intraoral radiograph of the left anterior maxillary teeth of the patient in 355. There has been cessation of growth of the permanent lateral incisor and canine as a result of radiotherapy.

357 This patient received external beam X-irradiation treatment to a sarcoma of the left parotid gland at age 5 years. There has been partial cessation of root growth and premature apical closure in all the permanent teeth. Despite this, all the permanent teeth had erupted into their correct occlusal position by the age of 11 years.

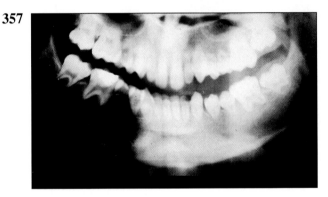

Self-mutilation

Factitious or artefactual lesions are seen in some disturbed or mentally handicapped patients; in patients with Lesch–Nyhan syndrome; in Gilles de la Tourette syndrome (tic, coprolalia and copropraxia); where there is sensory loss in the area; and where there is congenital indifference to pain (358) as in familial dysautonomia (Riley–Day syndrome).

Patients with epilepsy often suffer repeated orofacial trauma, causing soft tissue lacerations and scarring, and damage to teeth and/or jaws.

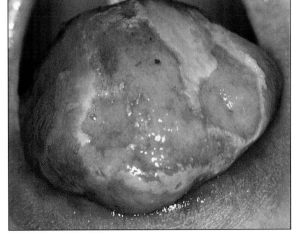

358 Erosion and scarring of the tip and dorsal surface of the tongue in a 3-year-old child with congenital insensitivity to pain. The tongue had been chewed between the upper and lower teeth. There was no intellectual impairment.

Syphilis

Oral lesions of acquired syphilis are rare in children. The primary chancre may affect the lip or tongue. Lesions of secondary syphilis (mucous patches (**359**) and snail track ulcers) can affect any intraoral site.

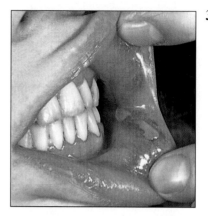

359

359 Mucous patches in secondary syphilis. N.B. Gloves should now always be worn during patient care.

Thrombocytopathy

Spontaneous gingival bleeding is often an early feature in platelet deficiencies or defects. Post-extraction bleeding may be a problem. Oral petechiae (**360**) and ecchymoses appear mainly at sites of trauma but can be spontaneous (**277, 279, 361**).

Petechiae therefore appear mainly in the buccal mucosa, on the lateral margin of the tongue, and at the junction of hard and soft palates.

Petechiae (**362**) and ecchymoses also appear readily on the skin, especially if there is trauma. Even the pressure from a sphygmomanometer can cause petechiae during the measurement of blood pressure.

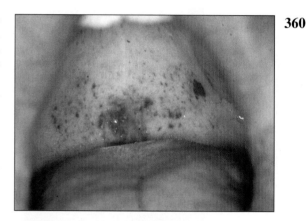

360

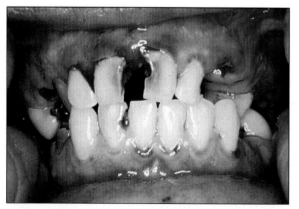

361

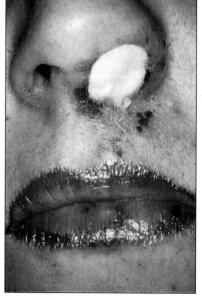

362

360 Oral petechiae in thrombocytopenia.

361 Spontaneous gingival bleeding in a teenage patient with idiopathic thrombocytopenic purpura who has a neglected dentition.

362 Petechiae are visible in the patient in **361** who has epistaxis, on the skin below the left nares, the lower lip and the chin.

Transplantation patients

Oral complications are common and can be a major cause of morbidity following bone marrow transplantation (BMT). Mucositis (**363**), infections, bleeding, xerostomia and loss of taste result from the effects of the underlying disease, chemo- or radio-therapy, and graft-versus-host disease (GVHD). The ventrum of the tongue, buccal and labial mucosa and gingiva may be affected by ulceration or mucositis.

The oral manifestations of acute GVHD have not been well documented but consist of painful mucosal desquamation and ulceration, and/or cheilitis, and the presence of lichenoid plaques or striae. Small white lesions (**364**) affect the buccal and lingual mucosa early on, but clear by day 14. Erythema and ulceration are most pronounced at 7–11 days after BMT, and may be associated with obvious infection. Oral candidosis is common, as is herpes simplex stomatitis (occasionally zoster), and there may be oral purpura.

The oral lesions in *chronic* GVHD are coincident with skin lesions, and include generalised mucosal erythema, lichenoid lesions, mainly in the buccal mucosa, and xerostomia with depressed salivary IgA levels in minor gland saliva. Xerostomia is most significant in the first 14 days after transplantation and is a consequence of drug treatment, irradiation and/or GVHD.

The chronic immunosuppression needed following organ transplantation predisposes to thrush and other infections. Some patients develop white lesions (keratoses) or hairy leukoplakia. Cyclosporin may induce gingival hyperplasia (**251, 365**). Rarely, oral malignant neoplasms have been recorded.

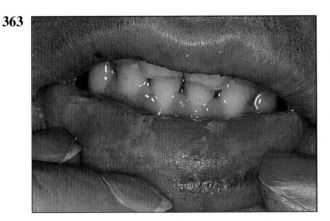

363 Labial ulceration and mucositis in bone marrow transplantation.

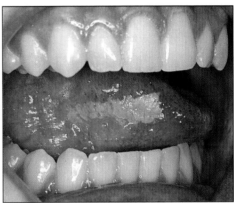

364 White patch in bone marrow transplant patient.

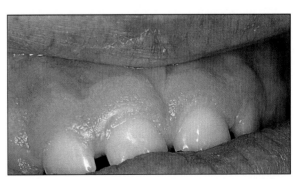

365 Early cyclosporin-induced gingival hyperplasia in a bone marrow transplant recipient.

Traumatic ulcers

366

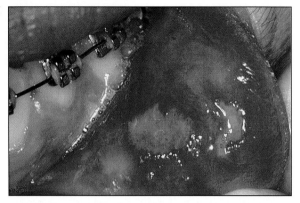

366 Oral ulceration caused by trauma from an orthodontic appliance.

Neonates occasionally develop an ulcer in the palate (Bednar's ulcer) which is thought may be caused by trauma from the examining finger of the paediatrician. Traumatic ulcers are common in children, usually caused by accidental biting, hard foods, appliances (**366**), or following dental treatment or other trauma. In child abuse (non-accidental injury), ulceration of the upper labial fraenum may follow a traumatic fraenal tear. Bruised and swollen lips, lacerated fraenae, and even subluxed teeth or fractured mandible can all be features of child abuse.

The lingual fraenum may be traumatised by repeated rubbing over the lower incisor teeth in children with recurrent bouts of coughing—as in whooping cough (termed Riga–Fedes disease) (**117**).

Varicella-zoster virus infections

Varicella (chickenpox) is a highly contagious herpes virus infection caused by the varicella-zoster virus (VZV). After an incubation period of 2–3 weeks, a variably dense rash appears, concentrated mainly on the trunk and head and neck (i.e. centripetal) (**367**). The typical rash goes through macular, papular, vesicular and pustular stages before crusting (**368**). The rash crops in waves over 2–4 days, so that lesions at different stages are typically seen.

The oral mucosa is commonly involved but there may be isolated lesions only. Vesicles appear (**369**), especially in the palate, and then rupture to produce painful round or ovoid ulcers with an inflammatory halo.

Maxillary or mandibular zoster (shingle) is rare in childhood but may then be associated with ipsilateral dental hypoplasia following the ulceration and rash.

367 Chickenpox: the rash is typically centripetal—on the trunk and face mainly.

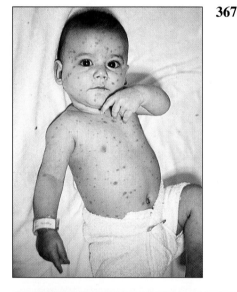

367

368

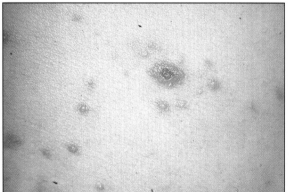

368 Chickenpox rash evolves from macules to papules, vesicles and pustules before scabbing.

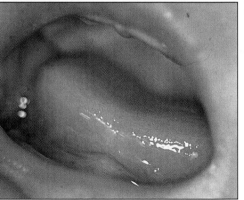

369

369 Oral vesiculation in chickenpox.

Vitamin deficiencies

Vitamin B deficiency is rare in children in the developed world. It may cause a sore mouth sometimes with ulcers or atrophic glossitis which presents as a depapillated and smooth tongue (**315, 316**). Red lines or red patches on the ventrum of the tongue (Moeller's glossitis) are fairly typical of early vitamin B_{12} deficiency. Oral ulcers and angular stomatitis are also common features (**370**). Angular stomatitis is seen particularly in vitamin B_{12} and in riboflavin deficiency. In Western countries, vitamin B_{12} deficiency is rarely dietary in origin but usually due to pernicious anaemia, gastric or small intestinal disease.

Deficiency of other haematinics (iron or folic acid) can also manifest (**371**) with glossitis (**372**), angular stomatitis and mouth ulcers. The most common cause of iron deficiency in Western countries is chronic haemorrhage but this is rare in children. Folic acid deficiency may be dietary.

When bone marrow iron stores are depleted, there is a stage of iron deficiency without anaemia (sideropenia) and before red cell changes are evident. Angular stomatitis and sore mouth are oral manifestations which may be seen in the pre-anaemic stage as well as in anaemia. Organic lesions are not always demonstrable though the mouth is sore.

Scurvy, with gingival swelling, is caused by vitamin C deficiency, but is rare.

370

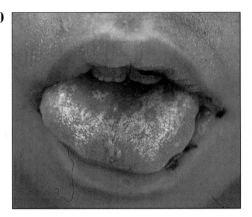

370 Tongue in pellagra showing ulceration.

371

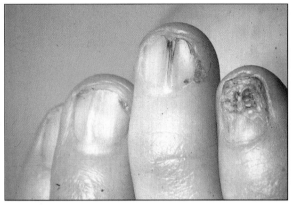

371 Iron deficiency in a 10-year-old child. Koilonychia is the term given to nail changes first evidenced by brittleness and dryness, later by flattening and thinning, and finally by concavity (spoon-shape). In addition, there is a chronic fungal infection of the nailbed of the index finger.

372

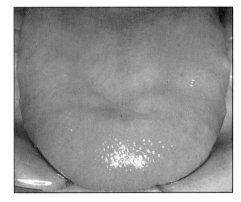

372 Chronic atrophic glossitis in the same child as **371**. There is some atrophy of the papillae and mucous membrane, giving the tongue a smooth glazed appearance. The atrophy begins at the edges and later affects the whole tongue. As a result the tongue appears moist and exceptionally clean.

6. Acquired Salivary Gland Disorders

Abnormal salivary flow

Few children complain of a dry mouth: most have more than adequate saliva. In true xerostomia, the dry mucosa may become tacky and the lips adhere one to another (**373**). An examining dental mirror may often stick to the mucosa. The main causes of dry mouth are iatrogenic, occasionally from drugs (those with anticholinergic or sympathomimetic activity), usually from irradiation of the salivary glands, or graft-versus-host disease.

Dehydration, as in diabetes, is an occasional cause. Rarely, there is salivary gland agenesis or disease of glands such as Sjögren's syndrome, sarcoidosis or HIV disease (**Table 11**).

Sialorrhoea (ptyalism) is more common and drooling is seen not infrequently in mentally handicapped children or those with poor control of the orofacial muscles, or where there are inflammatory oral lesions.

Table 11 Main causes of dry mouth in childhood.
IATROGENIC
Drugs with anticholinergic effects
Atropine and analogues
Tricyclic antidepressants
Antihistamines
Antiemetics
Phenothiazines
Drugs with sympathomimetic effects
Ephedrine and other decongestants
Bronchodilators
Amphetamines and appetite suppressants
Radiotherapy
Graft-versus-host disease
DEHYDRATION
Diabetes mellitus
Diarrhoea and vomiting
ORGANIC DISEASE OF GLANDS
Sjögren's syndrome
Sarcoidosis
HIV infection
Agenesis
PSYCHOGENIC
Anxiety states
Depression
Hypochondriasis

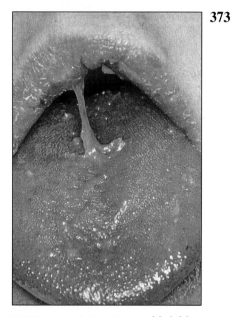

373

373 Xerostomia in a 4-year-old child as a result of complete agenesis of the major salivary glands. The dry mucosa is very tacky with strands of thick mucoid saliva. Agenesis was confirmed by a technetium pertechnetate radionuclide scan.

Mucoceles

Most mucoceles are caused by saliva extravasating into the tissues from a damaged salivary duct (extravasation cysts) and are seen in the lower labial (**374**) and ventral lingual mucosa. Occasional mucoceles are retention cysts.

The mucocele is a dome-shaped, fluctuant, bluish, non-tender, submucosal swelling with a normal overlying mucosa. A few arise within the epithelium and such superficial mucoceles appear as small vesicles.

Mucoceles arising from the sublingual gland are termed ranulas, because of their resemblance to a frog's belly (**375**). Rarely, a ranula extends through the mylohyoid muscle—a plunging ranula.

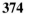
374

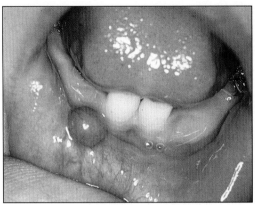

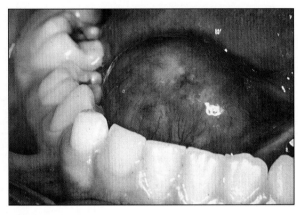
375

374 Mucocele in a common site, the lower lip.

375 A ranula of the right sublingual gland with the classic bluish translucent appearance said to resemble the belly of a frog.

Sialolithiasis and sialadenitis

Salivary calculi (sialoliths) are uncommon in children. They usually affect the submandibular duct, are sometimes asymptomatic, but may present with pain in, and swelling of, the gland—particularly around mealtimes. Calculi are usually yellow or white and can sometimes be seen in the duct or may be palpable. Not all are radio-opaque.

Stones are even less common in the parotid and less often radio-opaque. Obstruction of any gland can also be caused by mucus plugs, strictures, or the oedema associated with ulceration of the duct papilla.

Mumps (**376, 377**) is an acute infection with the mumps virus and predominantly affects the major salivary glands. Coxsackie, echo-, and other viruses occasionally cause similar features.

The incubation period of 2–3 weeks is followed by fever, malaise and sialadenitis, which can affect not only mainly the parotids but also the submandibular glands. The most obvious intraoral feature is swelling and redness at the duct orifice of the affected gland (papillitis). There is tender swelling with trismus. This may be unilateral but is more frequently bilateral. Pancreatitis, oophoritis and orchitis are less common features.

Suppurative parotitis (**378**) may occur as primary disease or as a complication of parotitis due to another cause. It is usually unilateral and presents with fever, pain and a swollen and tender parotid gland.

Recurrent parotitis (**379**) is an idiopathic parotid swelling that may be seen in otherwise healthy children. It is usually unilateral but may occur simultaneously or alternately on the contra-lateral side. Most cases appear related to congenital duct anomalies. There is little pain, and the salivary swelling lasts 2–3 weeks with spontaneous regression. Usually the condition resolves after puberty. The salivary gland disease of HIV infection is shown on p. 80 (**270**). Causes of swelling of salivary glands are shown in **Table 12**.

376

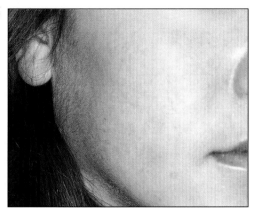

376 Mumps parotitis.

377

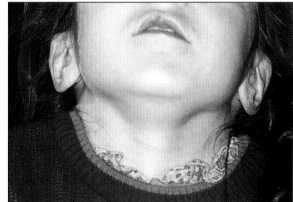

377 Mumps; bilateral parotitis and left submandibular sialadenitis.

Table 12 Main causes of salivary gland swelling in childhood.

LOCAL

Inflammatory	(Ascending bacterial sialadenitis)
Duct obstruction	(Usually by a calculus)
Neoplasms	(Various)

SYSTEMIC

Inflammatory	Mumps
	Recurrent parotitis
	HIV infection
	Sjögren's and sicca syndrome
	Sarcoidosis
	Actinomycosis
Others	Mikulicz's disease (lymphoepithelial lesion and syndrome)
	Chlorhexidine and other drugs
	Cystic fibrosis
	Sialosis (rarely)

378

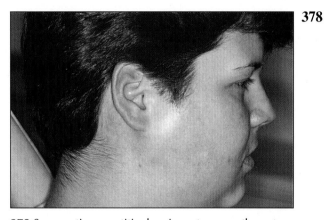

378 Suppurative parotitis showing a tense erythematous swelling.

379

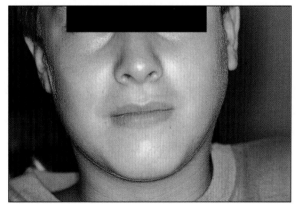

379 Recurrent parotitis.

Salivary neoplasms

380

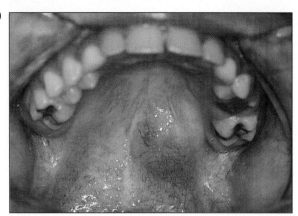

Salivary neoplasms are very rare in children, but usually involve the parotid. Most malignant neoplasms are mucoepidermoid tumours: most others are pleomorphic salivary adenomas (**380**).

380 Pleomorphic salivary adenoma in palatal glands in a 12-year-old child.

7. Acquired Musculoskeletal Disorders

Fibrous dysplasia

Fibrous dysplasia (**381**) (*see also* Cherubism, p. 12) is an uncommon benign fibro-osseous lesion, of unknown aetiology. The swelling is painless and typically stops growing at the time of skeletal maturity.

Four subgroups of fibrous dysplasia have been described: the most common is involvement of one bone (monostotic) (**382**): there is also polyostotic fibrous dysplasia; polyostotic fibrous dysplasia of Albright's syndrome; and a form confined to the craniofacial complex (craniofacial fibrous dysplasia) (**383**).

The typical appearance on radiography is of a 'ground glass' pattern (**384**). Bone scan using technetium diphosphonate shows increased uptake of radionuclide in fibrous dysplasia.

Albright's syndrome (McCune–Albright syndrome) is the association of polyostotic fibrous dysplasia with cutaneous hyperpigmentation (**385**), precocious puberty and occasionally other endocrine disorders.

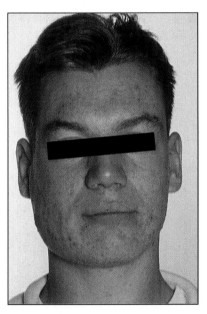

381 Fibrous dysplasia affecting the right side of the mandible in a teenager.

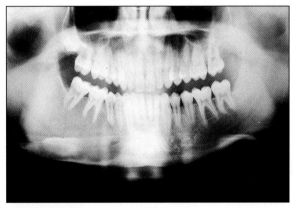

382 There is marked asymmetry with bony expansion on the affected side in the patient in **381**. The radiograph shows the typical 'ground glass' appearance replacing normal trabecular architecture. The roots of the teeth are unaffected by the bony changes.

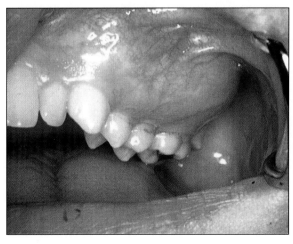

383 Typical maxillary alveolar expansion in fibrous dysplasia.

384

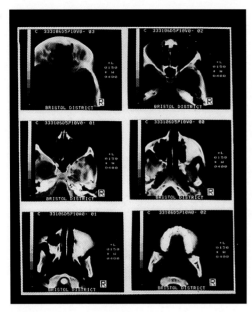

384 Fibrous dysplasia demonstrated on a CT scan.

385

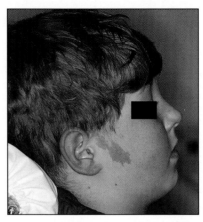

385 Skin hyperpigmentation in Albright's syndrome.

Masseteric hypertrophy

The masseter hypertrophies especially where there are parafunctional habits such as jaw-clenching or bruxism. There is unilateral or bilateral masseteric enlargement (**386, 387**) and sometimes a little tenderness in the affected muscle.

386

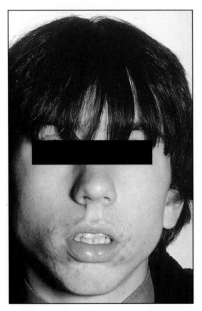

387

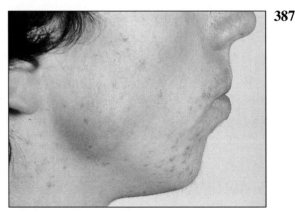

386, 387 Bilateral masseteric hypertrophy.

Odontogenic cysts and tumours

Odontogenic cysts and tumours are rare in children, though odontomes are not (*see* p. 66). Periapical dental cyst is the most common odontogenic cyst. Ameloblastoma is the most common tumour, is usually seen in an adolescent, and typically involves the region around the angle of the mandible (**388, 389**).

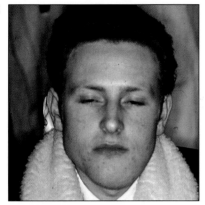

388 Ameloblastoma in right mandible.

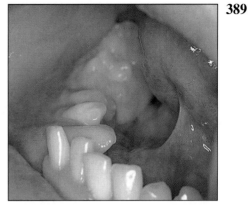

389 Ameloblastoma in the patient in **388**, showing tooth displacement.

Temporomandibular joint disorders

Arthritis

Pyogenic arthritis of the temporomandibular joint (TMJ) is rare but may follow a penetrating injury; may result from contiguous infection; or may be haematogenous, for example, gonococcal. Infection of the TMJ may result in ankylosis and impaired mandibular growth.

Juvenile rheumatoid arthritis (**390**) (20% of which is Still's syndrome with systemic disease) may also interfere with mandibular growth and cause ankylosis. Rheumatoid arthritis is a chronic relapsing inflammatory arthritis which usually affects many diarthrodial joints and is characterised by morning stiffness of the joints which, in advanced disease, become severely deformed. Osteoporosis, flattening of the mandibular condyle, marginal irregularities and limited movement may be seen. There may be restricted mouth opening.

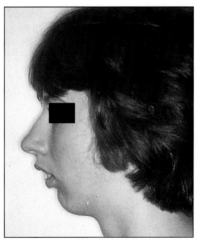

390 Juvenile rheumatoid arthritis has affected the temporomandibular joint and impaired mandibular growth, resulting in severe retrognathia.

Subluxation

Some other patients are able to sublux their TMJ deliberately. Subluxation is especially liable to occur in hypermobility syndromes, such as Ehlers–Danlos syndrome (*see* p. 23).

Temporomandibular pain-dysfunction syndrome (facial arthromyalgia) is a common complaint, characterised by discomfort, and/or clicking and/or locking of the TMJ. Seen predominantly in young adult females and rarely in children, the aetiology is unclear but may include psychogenic and/or occlusal factors. Clinical features include discomfort on palpation of the TMJ and masticatory muscles, occasional crepitus of the TMJ and limitation of mandibular movements. Plain radiographs of the TMJ are usually normal.

Pain-dysfunction syndrome of the TMJ may be associated with migraine and other disorders which have a psychogenic element.

Growth disorders

Impaired mandibular growth may be associated with generalised growth disorders, or where there is damage to the condylar growth centre—typically by infection or irradiation.

Generalised growth disorders such as acromegaly may lead to increased condylar growth, and prognathism.

Less defined are the causes of facial hemihyperplasia.

8. Other Relevant Lesions

Actinomycosis

Actinomycosis (**391**) is rare in children. It typically follows trauma and is seen over the mandibular region.

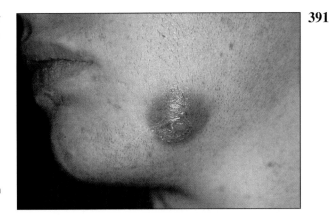

391 Actinomycosis showing the typical dusky purplish appearance at a common site.

Carcinoma

Oral carcinoma is extremely rare in children. Labial carcinoma (**392**) may be predisposed to by rare conditions such as xeroderma pigmentosum.

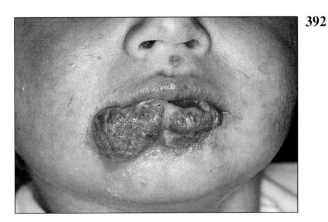

392 Carcinoma of the lip in a child.

Cat scratch disease

Cat scratch disease is caused by a small pleomorphic bacillus transmitted by cats, usually by a scratch, and typically affecting children. Three to 5 days after contact there is a papule which vesiculates and then heals. There may be fever and there is always tender regional lymphadenitis (**393**). Sometimes there is a rash or other complications.

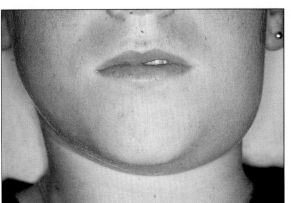

393 Cat scratch lymphadenitis affecting submandibular lymph nodes.

Cellulitis

Cellulitis (**394**) is rare. It is typically caused by infection with *Streptococcus pyogenes*.

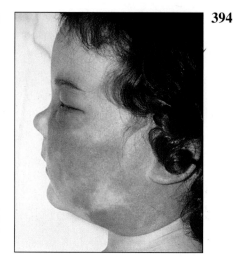

394

394 The erythema and swelling of facial cellulitis. Periorbital swelling has completely closed the left eye. The origin of this infection were carious left maxillary primary molars and a first permanent molar.

Cheilitis

Cheilitis may be caused by various factors, including excess sunlight exposure (**395**), drugs such as etretinate, chemical or other burns, or by allergies. Children may develop a habit of licking the lip and adjacent skin, leading to some erythematous circumoral lesions (**396, 397**). Candidosis may infect some of these lesions.

Lip-biting is a common habit, particularly in anxiety states, and may be associated with a few traumatic petechiae.

Persistent scaling of the vermillion of the lips (exfoliative cheilitis) is seen mainly in adolescent or young adult females. It may have a somewhat cyclical nature but is of unknown, possibly factitious, aetiology. The lips scale and peel and can be covered with a shaggy yellowish coating.

Lip fissures (**398**) are fortunately uncommon. A fissure may develop in the lip where a patient, typically a child, is mouth breathing. Lip fissures are also common in Down's syndrome and the lips may also split if swollen, for example, in oral Crohn's disease or orofacial granulomatosis (**301**).

Cheilitis granulomatosa is an uncommon cause of lip swelling (**399, 400**).

395

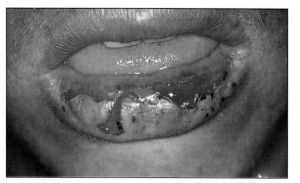

395 Actinic cheilitis after excessive exposure to tropical sun.

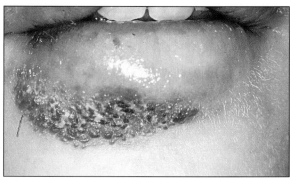

396

396 Lip-licking cheilitis affecting the lower lip.

397

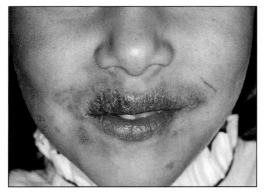

397 Lip-licking cheilitis affecting the upper lip.

398

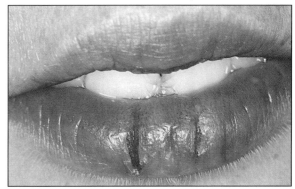

398 Lip fissure.

399

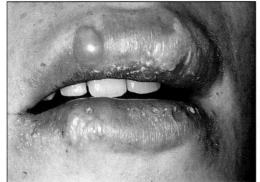

399 Acute exacerbation of cheilitis granulomatosa with diffuse swelling of the lips, scaling and vesicles/pustules on the vermilion border. Pain is not generally a feature of this condition.

400

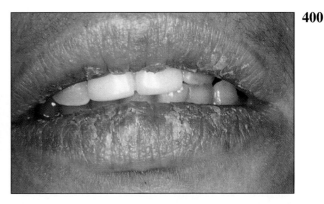

400 The appearance of the lips in patient in 399 in a relatively quiescent phase of cheilitis granulomatosa. This is a chronic condition of unknown aetiology which may persist for many years.

Facial palsy

Lower motor neurone paralysis of the facial (VIIth) nerve in a child or adolescent is usually due to Bell's palsy. Other causes may include head injury (401, 402), surgical damage or tumours. When asked to smile the patient is unable to raise the upper lip on the affected side.

401

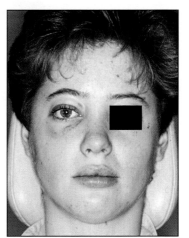

402

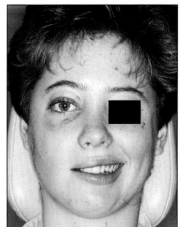

401, 402 Facial palsy resulting from a basal skull fracture on the right side in a road accident. There is residual periorbital haematoma on the right side, as well as the palsy.

Macroglossia

Macroglossia, a large tongue, is rare and typically occurs in children with congenital disorders—*see* **Table 13**.

Table 13 Main causes of macroglossia and microglossia in childhood.

MACROGLOSSIA

    Down's syndrome
    Beckwith–Wiedemann syndrome

MICROGLOSSIA

    Aglossia-adactylia syndrome
    Moebius' syndrome

Osteomyelitis

Osteomyelitis of the jaws is rare in children unless there is an immune defect (**403**). Neonates are occasionally afflicted by *Staphylococcus aureus* causing a maxillary osteomyelitis (**404**).

403

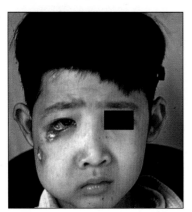

404

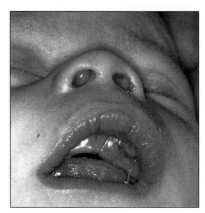

403 Maxillary osteomyelitis in a malnourished patient.

404 Maxillary osteomyelitis in a neonate.

Scleroderma

Scleroderma is rare in children but localised scleroderma (morphoea) may occasionally affect the face and lips (*en coup de sabre*) (**405**) and may extend intraorally. In contrast to classical scleroderma, there is no widening of the periodontal ligament.

405

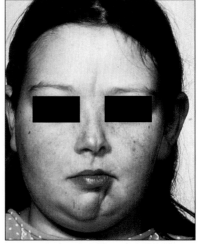

405 *En coup de sabre* in a girl.

9. Child Physical Abuse (Non-Accidental Injury—NAI)

A child is considered to be abused if he or she is treated in a way that is unacceptable in a given culture at a given time. The last two clauses are important because not only are children treated differently in different countries, but also within a country and even within a society there are sub-cultures of behaviour, and variations of opinion as to what constitutes abuse.

NAI is now recognised as an international issue. Each year at least 4000 children in the USA and 200 children in the UK will die as a result of abuse or neglect and more than 95% of serious intracranial injuries during the first year of life are said to be the result of abuse.

NAI encompasses all social classes, but more cases have been identified in the lower socio-economic groups. Many cases of NAI are by the child's parents or by persons known to the child. Often the mother of the affected child is divorced or single. It is also common for a cohabitant who is living in the home, but who is not related to the child, to be the perpetrator. Young parents, often of low intelligence, are more likely to be abusers, especially if they have been abused themselves during childhood. Contributing factors to abuse on behalf of the adults involved include drug and alcohol abuse, poverty, unemployment and marital problems. Children already at risk may add to the stress by continually crying, throwing tantrums or soiling their clothes. In addition, the child may be handicapped, be the result of an unwanted pregnancy or may fail to attain parental expectations.

NAI is not a full diagnosis, it is merely a symptom of disordered parenting. The aim of intervention is to diagnose and cure (if possible) the disordered parenting and prevent further injury. A significant proportion of abused children returned to the home environment without intervention will die or suffer serious re-injury.

The face is often the focus of impulsive violence and 50% of cases diagnosed as NAI have oro-facial trauma. Injuries can take the form of bruises, abrasions and lacerations, burns, bites, eye injuries, dental trauma and fractures. Accidental bruises usually involve skin overlying bony prominences and rarely affect the soft areas of the face. Inflicted bruises occur at typical sites (**406**) and fit recognisable patterns, e.g. slap marks on the cheek (**407**) or pinch marks on the ear (**408**). Bruising of the upper labial frenum of a young child can be produced by forcible bottle feeding. Intraoral burns and lacerations

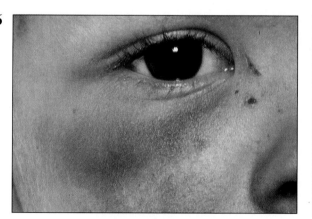

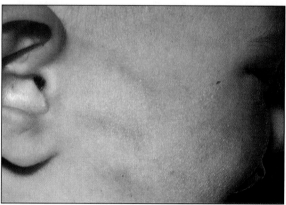

406 Bruising and small lacerations around the right eye. The bruising is of two different vintages. The blue black-areas are recent and the brown-yellow areas older.

407 Tram-line parallel marks on the cheek characteristic of a slap mark.

are usually caused by hot food/drink and the feeding implement respectively. Abrasions (**409**) and lacerations of the face and mouth (**410**) may be caused by a variety of objects, but are most commonly due to rings or fingernails on the inflicting hand. Burns from solid objects on the face are usually without blistering and the shape of the burn often resembles its agent. Cigarette burns (**411**) give circular punched out lesions of uniform size and are pathognomonic for child abuse. Techniques are now available to assist in bitemark identification. Fractures of the facial skeleton are relatively uncommon in child abuse cases, but are an indication for full skeletal radiographic survey which may show evidence of multiple fractures at different stages of healing.

The dental practitioner may be the first professional to suspect physical abuse as a result of injuries to the orofacial structures. The primary aim of all professionals involved is to ensure the safety of the child. The method of liaison and referral between dental practitioners and other health care professionals involved in NAI will vary in different localities depending on the guidelines issued by the local area Child Protection Unit.

408

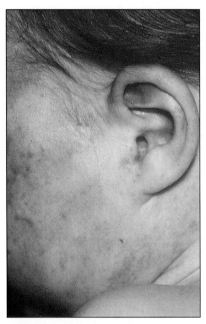

409

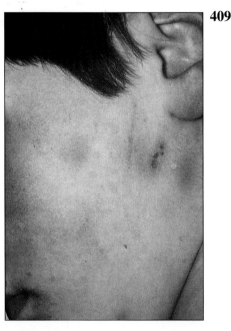

408 A pinch mark bruise of the ear and fading slap mark injuries of the cheek.

409 Bruising and abrasions of the cheek. The pattern was inconsistent with the explanation of an accidental injury.

410

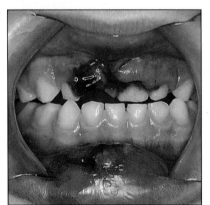

411

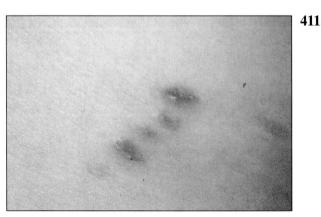

410 Injury to the primary teeth, upper gingiva and lower lip due to blunt trauma.

411 Well-circumscribed lesions characteristic of cigarette burns shown here on a child's back.

Further Reading

Abrams R.G. & Josell S.D. The role of the pediatrician in oral health care (1991). *Pediatr. Clin. N. Amer.*, **38**: 1049–1087.

Braham R.L. Oral soft tissue lesions in children and adolescents (1984). *The Practitioner*, **228**: 319–325.

Callender D.L., Robert A. & Frankenthaler M.D. Salivary gland neoplasms in children (1992). *Arch. Otolaryngol. Head Neck Surg.*, **118**: 472–476.

Cooley R.O. & Sanders B.J. The pediatrician's involvement in prevention and treatment of oral disease in medically compromised children (1991). *Pediatr. Clin. N. Amer.*, **38**: 1265–1287.

Dilley D.C., Siegel M.A. & Budnick S. Diagnosing and treating common oral pathologies (1991). *Pediatr. Clin. N. Amer.*, **38**: 1227–1263.

Griffen A.L. & Goepferd S.J. Preventive oral health care for the infant, child and adolescent (1991). *Pediatr. Clin. N. Amer.*, **38**: 1209–1226.

Johnsen D.C. The role of the pediatrician in identifying and treating dental caries (1991). *Pediatr. Clin. N. Amer.*, **38**: 1173–1207.

Josell S.D. & Abrams R.G. Managing common dental problems and emergencies (1991). *Pediatr. Clin. N. Amer.*, **38**: 1325–1350.

Kaufman F.L. Managing the cleft lip and palate patient (1991). *Pediatr. Clin. N. Amer.*, **38**: 1127–1147.

Luker J. & Scully C. Paediatric oral medicine. 1. Soft tissue lesions of the face and neck (1987). *Dental Update*, **14**: 391–399.

Luker J. & Scully C. Paediatric oral medicine. 2. Bony lesions and deformities of the face (1988). *Dental Update*, **15**: 15–25.

Luker J. & Scully C. Paediatric oral medicine. 3. The teeth (1988). *Dental Update*, **15**: 108–134.

Luker J. & Scully C. Paediatric oral medicine. 4. The gingiva (1988). *Dental Update*, **15**: 198–201.

Luker J. & Scully C. Paediatric oral medicine. 5. The oral mucosa (i) (1988). *Dental Update*, **15**: 292–298.

Luker J. & Scully C. Paediatric oral medicine. 5. The oral mucosa (ii) (1988). *Dental Update*, **15**: 370–373.

Poole A.E. & Redford-Badwal D.A. Structural abnormalities of the craniofacial complex and congenital malformations (1991). *Pediatr. Clin. N. Amer.*, **38**: 1089–1125.

Porter S.R. & Scully C. Primary immunodeficiency. In: Oral Manifestations of Systemic Disease. 2nd edition. Eds: Jones J.H. & Mason D.K., Balliere Tindall, London, 1990, pp. 112–161.

Porter S.R. & Scully C. Radiograph Interpretation in Dentistry. Oxford University Press, Oxford, 1991.

Scully C. & Flint S. Atlas of Stomatology. Martin Dunitz, London, 1989.

Scully C. The Mouth and Perioral Tissues in Health and Disease. Heinemann, Oxford, 1989.

Scully C., Porter S.R. & Greenspan D. Secondary immunodeficiency. In: Oral Manifestations of Systemic Disease. 2nd edition. Eds: Jones J.H. & Mason D.K., Balliere Tindall, London, 1990, pp. 162–182.

Scully C. The oral cavity. In: Textbook of Dermatology. 5th edition. Eds: Champion R.H., Burton J. & Ebling F.J.G., Blackwells, Oxford, 1991, pp. 2689–2769.

Smith R.J. Identifying normal and abnormal development of dental occlusion (1991). *Pediatr. Clin. N. Amer.*, **38**: 1149–1171.

Welbury R.R. Child physical abuse. In: Traumatic Injuries of the Teeth. 3rd edition. Ed. Andreasen J.O. Munksgaard, Copenhagen, 1993, in press.

Index

Numbers in normal print are page numbers; numbers in bold print refer to illustrations.